I0479210

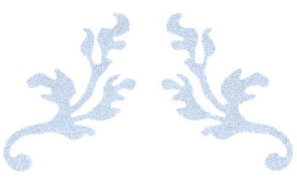

TRINITY OF HUMAN BEINGS

The Trinity within: A Journey to understand the Divinity in Ourselves

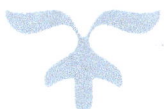

2023

OLGA FERRER ROCA

Barcelona (Spain)

Content

INTRODUCTION

Haven't you ever though on the analogy of the Trinity, 3 persons in one, Father-Son-Holy Spirit. Is there any other religion with that mystery? Does it make sense?

No, it doesn't until I began to understand myself. Until I began to think that we are created to the similarity of God. Until I admire my perfection as a human being. Until I realized that we are the Trinity: Mind-Body-Soul.

Then I started to realize which part belong to the mystery of God. Who is the Father? Should it be my conscious mind? Who is the Son? No doubt it is my body. Who is the Holy Spirit? Only the Soul is left, there is where we found our believes and our inspiration, should be the Spirit, our unconscious mind.

This book is devoted to show your divinity, to show your Trinity, to gain the Liberation in which Mind, Body and Soul get connected and you face the reality of God.

After you understand your Trinity, you will get convinced that you are never alone, your unconsciousness (your spirit, your soul...) is always with you, guiding you with its INTUITION.

God forgive me, forgive me to have the arrogance to show we are the Trinity. It is not a mystery anymore; it is just a storytelling that allow us to understand ourselves. Let's start.

The analogy of the Trinity is not a concept found in other major religions, but some belief systems may have similar concepts or ideas of multiple aspects of a deity or divine being. The idea that humanity is created in the image of God and therefore, we are also a Trinity of mind, body, and soul is an interpretation and personal belief that some shamanic religious also share. The author believes that understanding this concept can lead to a greater understanding of oneself and our communion with God.

The intention of this book is to better understand ourselves. Therefore, where the science has not arrived yet, I propose to see you inside, watching your own behavior. For that purpose, we have to use a storytelling that bring those concepts close to you, reading the book you have to dream, to get trapped, to feel... That is all about, it is not a scientific book (although there is a lot of science behind) is a self-meditation tool.

On this regard, some statements although containing accurate information may not be entirely true because we have oversimplified human complexity in order that the reader can easily understand his/her own body.

After reading it I hope you could identify the activity of your Trinity (Mind-Body-Soul) in the role to reach your Liberation. You could understand that you are God that demand appreciation, respect, and love. That you must take care of your personal God as well as the others. It requires reverence, work, meditation, understanding...

> **The Wisdom of the Universe allows you to get the 4 goals of life: Bliss, Joy, Wealth, Liberation.**

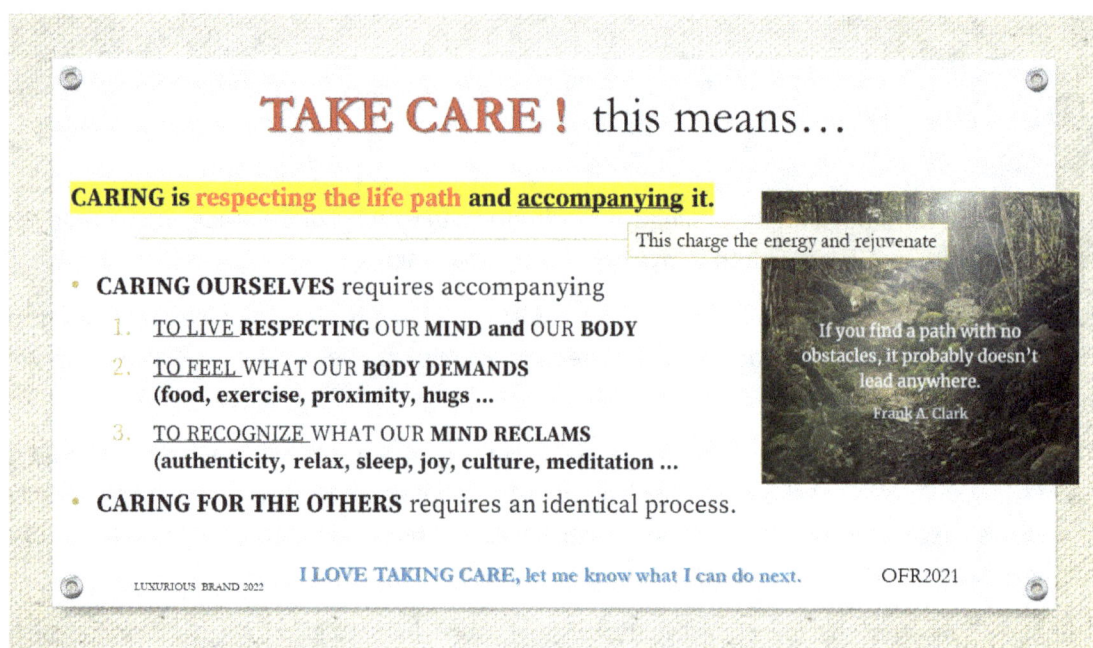

TAKE CARE ! this means…

CARING is respecting the life path and accompanying it.

- **CARING OURSELVES** requires accompanying
    1. TO LIVE **RESPECTING** OUR **MIND** and OUR **BODY**
    2. TO FEEL WHAT OUR **BODY DEMANDS** (food, exercise, proximity, hugs …
    3. TO RECOGNIZE WHAT OUR **MIND RECLAMS** (authenticity, relax, sleep, joy, culture, meditation …
- **CARING FOR THE OTHERS** requires an identical process.

This charge the energy and rejuvenate

If you find a path with no obstacles, it probably doesn't lead anywhere.
Frank A. Clark

LUXURIOUS BRAND 2022   I LOVE TAKING CARE, let me know what I can do next.   OFR2021

Noticed that in the content of the book images are as important as text, sometimes because they explain the text, sometimes include new knowledge, sometimes simplify …

It is not specifically stated, but CONSCIOUSNESS is a central core all over the book. You will learn that there are different type of consciousness including the unconsciousness, that the consciousness has evolved during human evolution and that our goal as Human Beings is to reach our Consciousness Liberation.

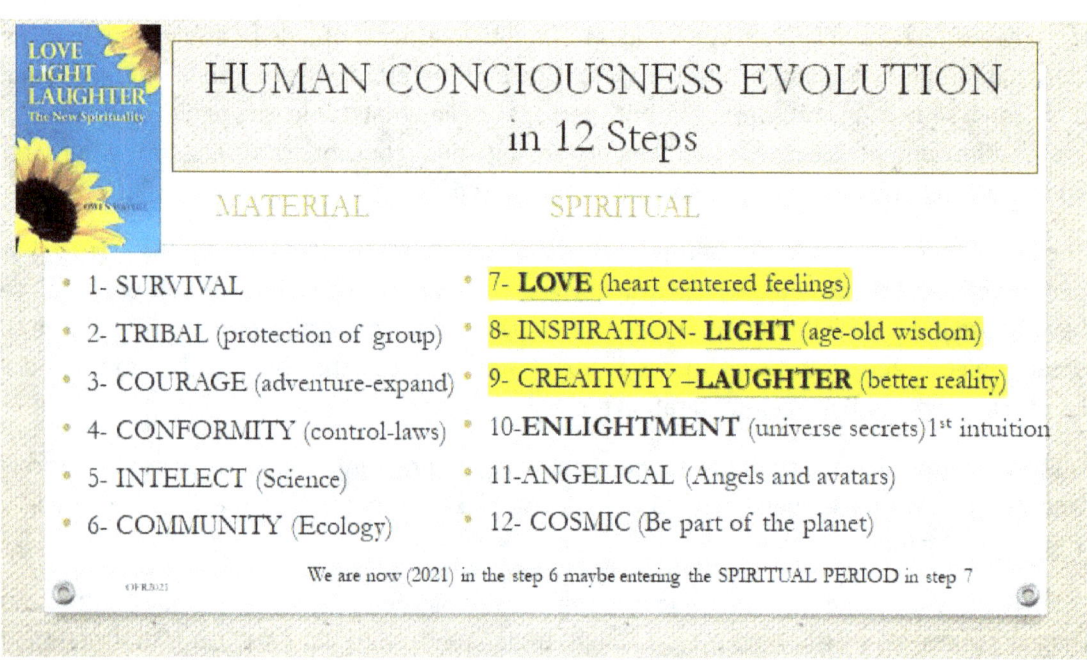

LOVE LIGHT LAUGHTER
The New Spirituality

HUMAN CONCIOUSNESS EVOLUTION in 12 Steps

MATERIAL	SPIRITUAL
1- SURVIVAL	7- **LOVE** (heart centered feelings)
2- TRIBAL (protection of group)	8- INSPIRATION- **LIGHT** (age-old wisdom)
3- COURAGE (adventure-expand)	9- CREATIVITY –**LAUGHTER** (better reality)
4- CONFORMITY (control-laws)	10-ENLIGHTMENT (universe secrets)1st intuition
5- INTELECT (Science)	11-ANGELICAL (Angels and avatars)
6- COMMUNITY (Ecology)	12- COSMIC (Be part of the planet)

We are now (2021) in the step 6 maybe entering the SPIRITUAL PERIOD in step 7

OFR2021

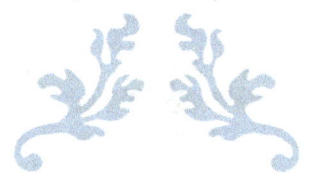

HOW IT STARTED

Everything started trying to study and understand self-hypnosis. Trying to understand why we are 50% of the time in self-hypnosis and that this is healthful for our mind and our body.

HYPNOSIS-1

You are probably aware that **50% of the time we are in a hypnotic state**. The good and outstanding performances (acting, playing music, dancing, driving, writing, teaching, athletics, public speaking, good reading ...) are only done under **self-hypnotic state**. The feeling of extreme happiness, euphoria, ... appear under self-hypnosis. In general, any concentration state in which surroundings disappear and the inner side is manifested, is a hypnotic state. And only when a performance is capable to induce an extreme focus (a hypnotic state) in others, we can reach their inner side. Unfortunately, there are no distinction between good and evil, Hitler or Rasputin hypnotic influence was equally effective. Nevertheless, hypnosis or hypnotic state is not the same as **hypnotic trance;** when one reaches the level of "trance" becomes sensitive to a given suggestions (the so-called *posthypnotic commands*). Although, keep in mind that nothing can be suggested to be done against our own will.

> Let's start by defining HYPNOSIS: It is a **highly focused state of mind** producing an altered state of consciousness, self or hetero induced (although all hypnosis is self-hypnosis), which manifests psychological and physiological changes due to the decay or disappearance of the conscious state **with the raise or appearance of the unconscious mind.**

- The conscious mind can only **deal with 7 to 9 items (bytes) of information** at any given time (*very few*). It is bombarded by 5 times as many upstream connections from our "animal brain" (in charge of survival and emotions) for each single downstream connection. Reason why, survival and emotions influence so much our conscious mind decisions.
- The unconscious mind is everything that is **happening in the background of our mind.** It works automatically without any conscious help, and it can **handle millions of pieces of data** all at the same time. The unconscious mind is also where our "innate creativity lies" and our **ability to imagine** big bold dreams. It's also where all our memories are stored (*2.5 petabytes=300 years of TV shows*). It is obvious that to reach this massive unconscious information we need **our all/maximum focus of attention.** Therefore, hypnosis is a hyper focused or hyper concentrated state into our subconscious mind, indeed into our Soul.

The unconscious is supposed to be in the non-dominant hemisphere (generally the right), and it is functioning **uncritically, timeless, holistic, inductive, symbolic, and integrative.** Our unconscious mind is not affected by the criticism, deduction, temporary and biased logics that guide our rational hemisphere, the dominant one (generally the left). And if the right side is the feminine and the left where main masculine attribute resides, dominant right hemisphere people (female, artist, poets...even left-handed people) do live in state of hypnosis much more often than the rest of people. *They live in connection, in communion, with their souls.*

> In fact, intuition, muses, inspiration, solving problems stages... are hypnotic states.

One of the classic **problem-solving hypnotic states** is the transition between awake and sleep. This is an essential period for researchers, mathematicians, innovators, inventors, creators, solution finders, solving problems of average people. At that moment our subconscious mind is predominant, but our conscious mind still is capable to question and guide us through the problem. It is our subconscious mind who answers by finding/creating solutions, using for this its massive pool of information gathered in years (as much pertinent this previous information is, as quicker the solution will be found).

Take advantage of this ability but never violate the rules of prudence or justice.

Creativity, therefore, is reduced to clearly present a problem to our mind (imagining it, visualizing it, supposing it, meditating it, contemplating it) to be able to create/invent an idea, concept, notion, or scheme along new unconventional lines. These is always better done in the sleep-awake transition.

Another good reason to avoid the insomnia and sleep sufficient hours.

Scientists say that the sleep N1 phase (at the beginning when dreams are dominated by brain *Theta-waves* linked to short-term memory) is the essential one. Not for me, that is at the end, in the awakening process, where I find my productivity, in the so-called "wet dreams", where "lucid dreams" are easier to handle and modify particularly for onironauts (people trained in lucid dreams).

Both can produce *post-hypnotic commands,* meaning elaborate suggestions that are given to us during **the sleeping hypnotic trance** and that therefore we will carry it out awake, always formulating a rational explanation for them. Those are an essential part of our mechanism of **problem-solving and discovering**.

In the Hypnosis-2 you will meet some of the brain waves listed below that directly may influence your everyday work.

Beta waves (14-30 Hz)

* Linear, externally directed left-brain thinking
* Associated with stress, anxiety and fear.
* Unsynchronized waves
* Useful for short term memory and routine jobs.

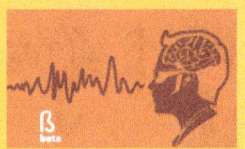

Alpha waves (8-13.9 Hz)

* Relaxed focus and good health
* Mental coordination
* Long-term memory
* Creativity and visualization.
* Associated with light meditation.

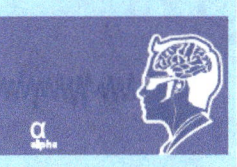

Theta waves (4-7.9 Hz)

* Reduced consciousness
* Deep meditation, intuition
* Vital for learning & memory
* High creativity, flashes of insight and inspirations.
* Spontaneous healing

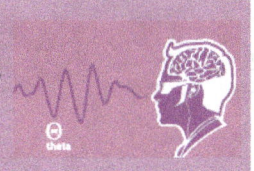

Delta waves (1-3.9 Hz)

* Deep sleep, unconsciousness
* Growth hormone released
* Loss of body awareness.
* Deep physical relaxation.
* Access to collective unconscious mind.

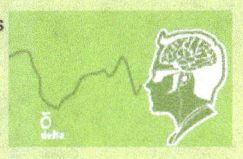

Genius Brain waves

Gamma waves (40 to 200/sec)

* Genius brain waves
* Higher level of consciousness.
* Experienced by monks & visionaries.
* Mystical experiences and out of body experiences.
* Hyper concentration & focus
* Crucial for "Self awareness & insight.

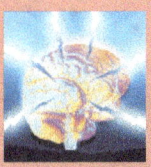

Epsilon waves (below 0.5 Hz)

* Experienced in very deep and advanced states of meditation
* Ecstatic states of consciousness
* High-level inspiration and creation.
* Spiritual insight and out-of-body and mystical experiences.

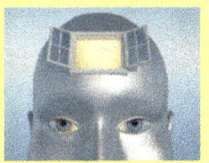

Human Brain Wave (thebrainwaves.org)

Our body may be totally renewed in 7-10 years. In ten years, we become a totally different person because all our cells have been changed, except for our partial conscious and all subconscious memory (our soul). i.e. the tongue taste buds get replaced every 10 days but the memory of the delicious taste of food you already knew or the new one you experience remains forever, stored in the memory sprouts of your brain neurons.

And **when we born**, our subconscious mind contains, coded in our DNA, the ancestors and heritage memories built and stored in our primitive neuron sprouts (in our soul) modified in the womb by mother hormones and our own hormone system. No doubt about it, it is the same coded DNA containing our evolution from oviparous (reptile fully form at birth) to mammals and there, from marsupials to placentals to protect our immature born imprints which complexity cannot be fully settle in just 9 months. The same coded DNA that with one extra chromosome erase evil in the mongolian children with trisomy 21.

As you can see, we are MORE than enough. Is there any doubt that we are holding **the Wisdom of the Universe?** As such, anytime humans create something, a disjunctive appears: (1) either to be guided by the emotion as a humble baker, rooted in the passion to create every day the best possible bread for everyone or (2) to be guided by the Ego of the chef enchanted with his Michelin's star restaurant, and devoted to please outstanding clients.

INTENTION coming from *the Ego* is weak, you can achieve a lot with hard work, exact plans, and discipline, but by the time you do it you have heart disease, sexual impotency, drug addiction, and probably a divorce. INTENTION must come from *our Values* raised in our "soul profile" in "our spirit" to produce a true success.

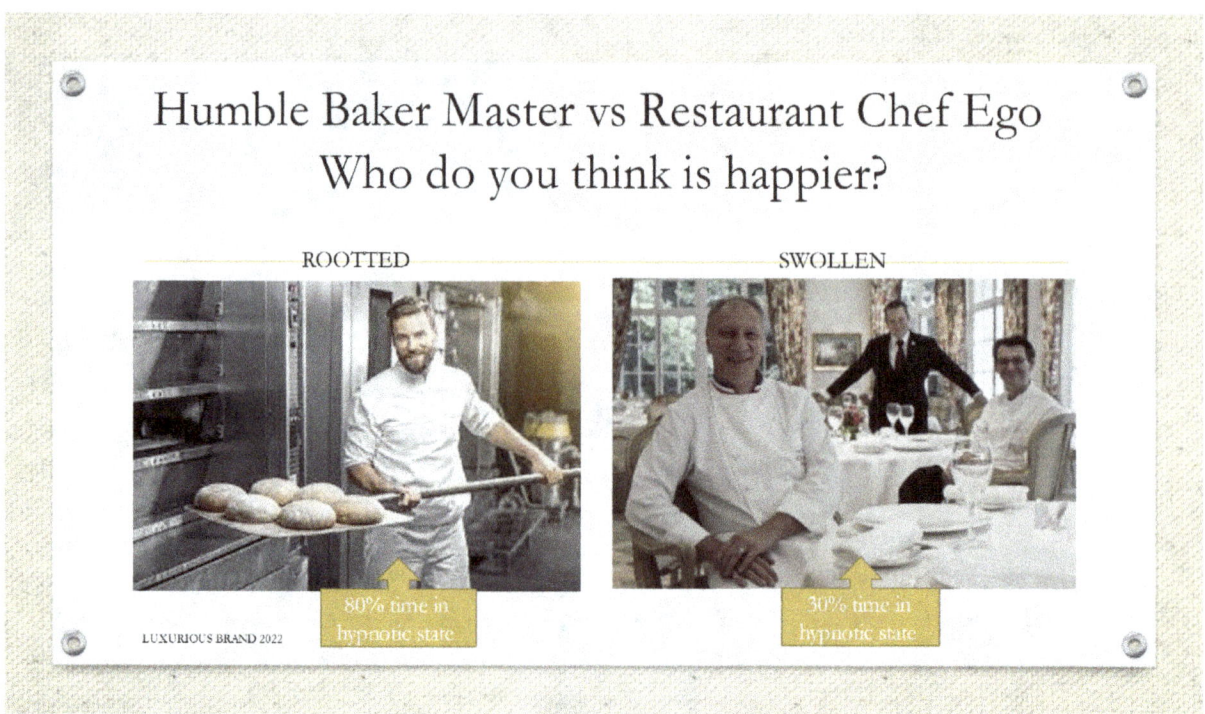

Humble Baker Master vs Restaurant Chef Ego
Who do you think is happier?

ROOTED   SWOLLEN

80% time in hypnotic state   30% time in hypnotic state

LUXURIOUS BRAND 2022

Who do you think is happier?

Who do you think have better **self-sense of accomplishment** when is alone?

In healthy cultures, no level of individual excellence justifies undermining people. We are not high performers if we do not elevate others. But bear in mind that for extremely sincere or passionate people, the **courtesy in treating** others is sometimes taken as a falsehood (Sting - the iconic rock music with an Introverted, Intuitive, Feeling, and Prospecting INFP-personality- is a good example). In contrast, **Vulnerability** according Brené Braum, from Houston University, is the point where love, the sense of belonging, courage, creativity, and joy are born. Vulnerability becomes necessary to establish deep links with our environment (we will cover it in the Mirror Neurons chapter).

Vulnerability is often seen as a key component in building trust and forming close relationships with others. The concept of mirror neurons is related to the ability of the brain to understand the actions, emotions and intentions of others, by simulating them internally. This is a key mechanism for the ability of empathy, which is a fundamental aspect of vulnerability.

Finally, to superficially approach the problem of the CONSCIOUNESS, you already know that when you get suggestions during an **hypnotic trance** this *posthypnotic commands* will be never against your own will, but you always "build" a story (you are a storyteller) that could justify your own behavior. Sperry explains very well how a consciousness story is build: In a patient with both hemispheres separated (girus cinguli cutted) if you give something (a bottle) to the left eye with an order (lift it up) this will go only to the right hemisphere; the patient will ask to the left hemisphere why I did this, the answer should have been "I do not know" but instead of this the patient build *a story to justify the action* (I am thirsty).

> Consciousness is a figurehead, an interpreter, a kind of narrator, who creates a story to explain in retrospect the inexplicable.

Pay attention in the way we are building our own life, our own reality, we are the creators. Now is clearer that this reality is different from one to another.

Consciousness acts as a mediator, creating a narrative to explain our actions and experiences. Our consciousness creates our own reality, which is unique and subjective to each individual. This highlights the idea that we are the creators of our own life and reality.

Even considering controversial that our reality is "entirely" subjective and unique to each individual, it has been shown that our perception and interpretation of reality is "strongly" influenced by our individual experiences and biases. And furthermore, that our consciousness is a storytelling builder.

This gives us another approach, stories reach quicker our consciousness, a storyteller can easier pierce the shell and enter directly into the consciousness. For this reason, religions in general are built over parables, in other word they teach us with stories to be able to reach our consciousness. In the chapter of The Verb, we will learn how momentous this is, it approaches us to God, since we are the only species capable to talk.

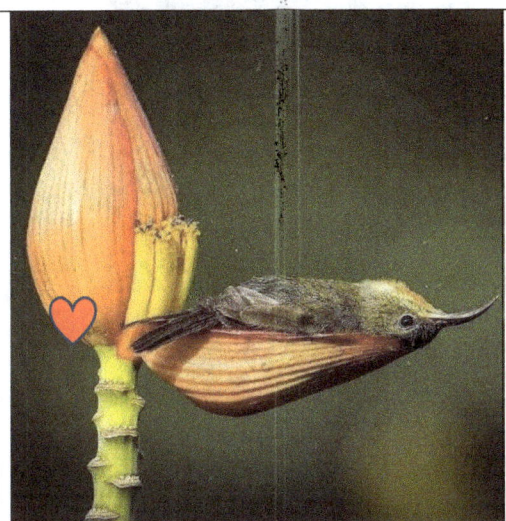

Program a healthy work-life,

care of excessive risks,

never succumb to guilt or shame. (depression)

Move from fear to love and

from the state of "doing"

to the state of "being".

Know yourself to be **strong** and

accept yourself to become invincible.

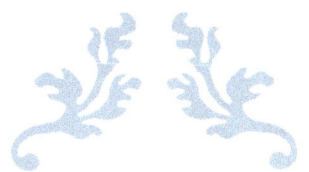

The influence of Hypnosis in the brain is very impressive and it is essential for Success.

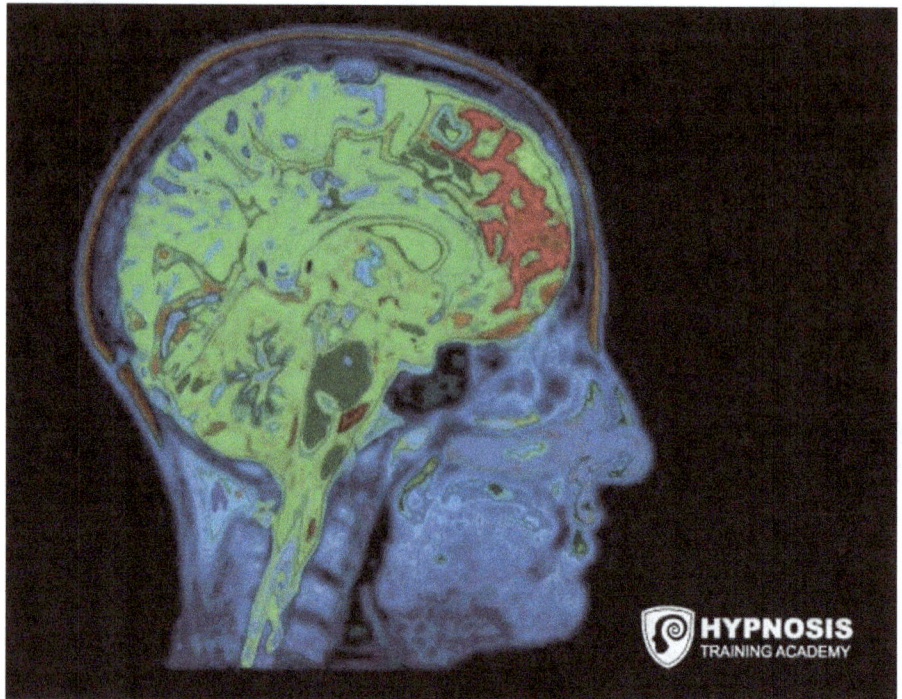

What is happening in the brain under hypnosis:
- Less activity in the dorsal anterior cingulate (making the brain **more relaxed and worry-free**)
- More <u>activity in</u> the brain area responsible for **<u>planning and organization</u> (frontal area, the intelligence area, the soul area)**
- Less activity in the part of the brain concerned with self-reflection (making people **<u>less inhibited</u> and less self-conscious**)

If you take into consideration what we said Hypnosis-1 about Lucid Dreams, you will understand that onironauts have a big prefrontal area. The pre-frontal cortex oversees the conscious cognitive processes, directly linked with the auto reflexive capability. Those people have therefore a specific ability to talk with his unconscious side, to connect mind and soul, to connect conscious and unconscious mind.

➢ One classical lucid hypnotic stage is acting. In these circumstances is very relevant to protect the subconscious mind, not to destroy the inner equilibrium in **the hypnotic process of <u>acting</u>** as could happens in difficult or extreme scenes (i.e. the actual Netflix series of "Euphoria" by Zendaya in which some of the actresses required medical rehabilitation, in spite that they hug and kiss each other -oxytocin shot- after difficult, stressful/cortisol scenes). Also, you probably understand why actors prefer theater to movies; not only by the close feed-back of public that raise their dopamine (as explain in the dopaminergic life), but by the prolong hypnotic state being "on stage" without interruptions (as the Master Baker, this could create a state of concentration that relax body and mind and/or reach the "Team Flow Level" synchronizing brains, temporal *Beta and Gamma brain waves* in the whole company or group of people).

> The **curative effect** of drama performance in individual problems is hypnosis-linked, allowing subconscious mind to manifest. Also, mirror neurons stimulation in good performances, is a self-hypnotic state, reaching in some cases the level of hypnotic trance allowing to suggest changes in the audience. Bear in mind the importance of **a good and ethical storyteller**: because when we start watching TV, we enter in a day-dream state, with restful *Alpha waves* slowing down approaching hypnotic frequencies; and, falling asleep can be a **hypnotic trance** that finish awaking when TV programme ended. **Destructive effect** is also possible: Violence, aggression, or abandon -in films, in war, at home, in life- are emotions that enter through mirror neurons of the *girus cinguli* (interpreting emotions) and between 8-12y (adolescence) get stored in the *hypocampus* (memory) to spread towards the *hypothalamus* and *amygdalae* where they **get fixed live-long**, becoming a repeated behavior when adults (in a script form). Sufficient not to expose adolescents to violent games, movies, or behaviors. And an explanation of the extreme aberrant reactions of people capable to kill parents and offprints for the sole reason of being deprived of mobile or social networks.

(Similar mechanisms guide the fixation of money-scripts that we will study later)

> The role of **hypnosis in personal relationships**. After desensitization (achieved after 3 years around) from the high-dopamine level of the *falling-in-love* period, the hypnotic state is essential to maintain softhearted love. But daily life overactivity (chronopathy), prevents the required concentration to reach a hypnotic state. And only in hypnotic state, souls (inner self) could get connected through their subconscious minds. This level of concentration is also reach by admiration or by mirror neurons stimulation hypnosis. The reason we close the eyes kissing is because this movement (**eyes up and eyelids down**) is being fundamental to enter self-hypnosis and is identical when we start to sleep. In relationships, a *hypnotic shot* should follow by an *appreciation act* expressing what we like from our counterpart. **Appreciation is infective**.

> People use to say that a person is genuine when his/her behavior come from inside, from the subconscious mind, because is behaving in a hypnotic state of concentration (in the process/in people/in an individual) that allows to reach the inner side of the counterpart /public. This produces a "*glowing effect*" that is hypnotic, and the essential part of the "Presence" in the moment, one of the three principles that make people "irresistible" which are: presence, self-esteem, divine emotions.
> (*) passion= bring your heart in what you do.

Know what makes people/you irresistible

1. **PRESENCE** **IN THE MOMENT** (Experience life, relationships and environment. Spirit involved, not possible of being distracted, awareness, tone voice, attentive on what it is, life centered.) OF WHAT IT IS AND WHO IS IN FRONT OF YOU.

2. **SELF-ESTEEM** (True self power, fearless, immune to criticism, center in yourself beyond your self image, you feel beneath no one, you know who you are, what you want, what your skills are, how to use them .) YOU KNOW WHAT YOU CONTRIBUTE AND RECEIVE.

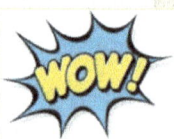

3. **DIVINE EMOTIONS** (Exude loving kindness, joy, compassion & equanimity) EMOTIONS IRRADIATED.

MAGNETIC- CHARMING- CHARISMATIC- ATTRACTIVE- IRRESISTIBLE- A LEADER

OFR 2019

➢ **Love your memories**, this is directly related to the "fan-phenomena" and your "love-life". To live in the past is not good, we have to live in the present; but loving memories, nice memories, bring us to the hypnotic state of happiness we had at that moment, and this is regenerative for our body allowing us to recover from stressful situations. Specifically, the "fan-phenomena" is in both directions: you with your fans, and your fans with you. Bring in mind your sensation before the pandemic, when you were able to connect with your fans' devotion in person. Erase the fear to your bad evil fans and keep the memory of your wonderful fans. Do the same with you love-life. Build a pool of good loving memories ready to be recalled neutralizing any stressful situation because when the stress is maintained in time has the risk to derive into depression.

➢ Hypnosis also play an important role in **good professors** or in **reading good books**. Yes, professors and books produce <u>an alter state of mind</u> with our imagination fully occupied at work and drawing all these evocated pictures into our mind (brain in *Gamma waves* state). We cannot put the book down because we are in hypnotic trance-like state, being immerse into the story or into the discovery or understanding of new things or processes that wonder us. That is the reason why we admire our good professors and see them "glowing".
   - Teaching requires the same hypnotic concentration because you must reach the soul of your pupils, you must open their minds, their intuition to the secrets of life and the universe, to allow them to think and create by themselves.

➢ And finally, it is easy to deduct that under the effect of psychotropic drugs as well as in **near-death** experiences where our <u>conscious brain disappears</u> (lower *Alpha waves*), we are capable to access and **review all our life** stored in our subconscious mind. At that moment, we are displaying brain waves like the hypnotic ones, particularly *Gamma waves* related to highly cognitive functions such as concentration, dreams, meditation, memory retrieval, conscious awareness, and those linked to memory flashbacks (attended visual stimulus). This is related with serotoninergic psychedelic chemicals (LSD or ayahuasca or endogenous **DMT- dimethyltryptamine**) influencing visual cortex. People think (not demonstrated yet) that a relevant source of endogenous DMT origin is the pineal gland, since it controls the sleep and therefore dreams. What we know is that DMT increase not only in brain but in all body under hypoxia (lack of oxygen) getting inactivated by the MAO enzyme as other Nervous System aromatic amines such as epinephrine, norepinephrine and **dopamine**.

Do you understand it? Did you like it? Every time you finish a work or get immerse in a renewal you should go to a hypnotic process to find yourself, what cares, what is your passion and your life meaning.

> Follow your purpose, in something you could create by your own.

We attract people with similar "inner values" (the ones you should discover) creating an appropriate ecosystem for success. Do not sacrifice yourself for your selfies, and don't confuse self-work by a network, because people with huge networks might have no self-work capable to bring them joy. Rediscover your purpose and regain your bliss. Live out of the FOMO (Fear Of Missing Out).

Never forget … YOU ARE ENOUGH, perfectly built to take care. Meaning, to reach the 4 goals in life DHARMA-KHAMA-ARTHA-MOKSHA: (1) Follow your purpose, your bliss; (2) Sensual delight through the 5 senses. Being mindful of every sense we experience, to become joyful (3) Currency (or wealth) a way we exchange our values. Our "soul profile" determine what our "inner values" are. When we exchange our inner values, we do currency (circulation) and exchanging currency is what money is. Therefore, you can generate a lot of money if you know what your values are, and you exchange with people those values (no other way is capable to bring wealth). (4) Achieve the Liberation, where the profound knowledge of yourself lets to see your mind, body, and soul directly connected and mutually influenced. We all are unique, we can't get the same type of liberation because our bodies require different ways to grow in mind, body, and soul.

I hope you enjoyed the knowledge and use it to storytelling your offprints. Our first task in education is "to shake life but leave it free to develop" and fair-tells are lies helping to understand life.

> Fight for your Self-esteem and include life acceptance and abandonment in the process.
>
> Self-esteem makes you feel fearless, independent of the good or bad opinions of the world, a winning recipe for success.

Do not translate the "law of attraction" as the majority do by "BE POSITIVE". Because it can be very stressful if you are not feeling positive, and it can exasperate others thinking you are pretending. The force comes from an **"AWAKEN MIND" open to resources such intuition or creativity.** Waking up is **about evolution**, is about acquiring higher consciousness, and reaching an infinite potential that belongs by nature to every human being. Intention *coming from the Ego* is weak, INTENTION must be born in *Your Values* the ones coming from your "soul profile" to be able to produce an invincible true success.

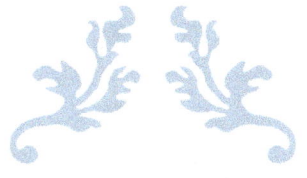

body and mind and/or reach the "Team Flow Level" synchronizing brains, temporal *Beta and Gamma brain waves* in the whole company or group of people).

> The **curative effect** of drama performance in individual problems is hypnosis-linked, allowing subconscious mind to manifest. Also, mirror neurons stimulation in good performances, is a self-hypnotic state, reaching in some cases <u>the level of hypnotic trance</u> allowing to suggest changes in the audience. Bear in mind the importance of **a good and ethical storyteller**: because when we start watching TV, we enter in a day-dream state, with restful *Alpha waves* slowing down approaching hypnotic frequencies; and, falling asleep can be a **hypnotic trance** that finish awaking when TV programme ended. **Destructive effect** is also possible: ==Violence, aggression, or abandon== -in films, in war, at home, in life- are emotions that enter through mirror neurons of the *girus cinguli* (interpreting emotions) and between 8-12y (adolescence) get stored in the *hypocampus* (memory) to spread towards the *hypothalamus* and *amygdalae* where they **get fixed live-long**, ==becoming a repeated behavior when adults== (in a script form). Sufficient not to expose adolescents to violent games, movies, or behaviors. And an explanation of the extreme aberrant reactions of people capable to kill parents and offprints for the sole reason of being deprived of mobile or social networks.

(Similar mechanisms guide the fixation of money-scripts that we will study later)

> The role of **hypnosis in <u>personal relationships</u>**. After desensitization (achieved after 3 years around) from the high-dopamine level of the *falling-in-love* period, the hypnotic state is essential to maintain softhearted love. But daily life overactivity (chronopathy), prevents the required concentration to reach a hypnotic state. And only in hypnotic state, souls (inner self) could get connected through their subconscious minds. This level of concentration is also reach by admiration or by mirror neurons stimulation hypnosis. The reason we close the eyes kissing is because this movement (**eyes up and eyelids down**) is being fundamental to enter self-hypnosis and is identical when we start to sleep. In relationships, a *hypnotic shot* should follow by an *appreciation act* expressing what we like from our counterpart. **Appreciation is infective**.

> People use to say that a person is genuine when his/her behavior come from inside, from the subconscious mind, because is behaving in a hypnotic state of concentration (in the process/in people/in an individual) that allows to reach the inner side of the counterpart /public. This produces a *"glowing effect"* that is hypnotic, and the essential part of the =="Presence"== in the ==moment==, one of the three principles that make people "irresistible" which are: presence, self-esteem, divine emotions.

    (*) passion= bring your heart in what you do.

Know what makes people/you irresistible

1. **PRESENCE IN THE MOMENT** (Experience life, relationships and environment. Spirit involved, not possible of being distracted, awareness, tone voice, attentive on what it is, life centered.) OF WHAT IT IS AND WHO IS IN FRONT OF YOU.

2. **SELF-ESTEEM** (True self power, fearless, immune to criticism, center in yourself beyond your self image, you feel beneath no one, you know who you are, what you want, what your skills are, how to use them .) YOU KNOW WHAT YOU CONTRIBUTE AND RECEIVE.

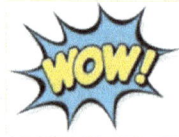

3. **DIVINE EMOTIONS** (Exude loving kindness, joy, compassion & equanimity) EMOTIONS IRRADIATED.

MAGNETIC- CHARMING- CHARISMATIC- ATTRACTIVE- IRRESISTIBLE- A LEADER

OFR 2019

➢ **Love your memories**, this is directly related to the "fan-phenomena" and your "love-life". To live in the past is not good, we have to live in the present; but loving memories, nice memories, bring us to the hypnotic state of happiness we had at that moment, and this is regenerative for our body allowing us to recover from stressful situations. Specifically, the "fan-phenomena" is in both directions: you with your fans, and your fans with you. Bring in mind your sensation before the pandemic, when you were able to connect with your fans' devotion in person. Erase the fear to your bad evil fans and keep the memory of your wonderful fans. Do the same with you love-life. Build a pool of good loving memories ready to be recalled neutralizing any stressful situation because when the stress is maintained in time has the risk to derive into depression.

➢ Hypnosis also play an important role in **good professors** or in **reading good books**. Yes, professors and books produce an alter state of mind with our imagination fully occupied at work and drawing all these evocated pictures into our mind (brain in *Gamma waves* state). We cannot put the book down because we are in hypnotic trance-like state, being immerse into the story or into the discovery or understanding of new things or processes that wonder us. That is the reason why we admire our good professors and see them "glowing".

  - Teaching requires the same hypnotic concentration because you must reach the soul of your pupils, you must open their minds, their intuition to the secrets of life and the universe, to allow them to think and create by themselves.

➢ And finally, it is easy to deduct that under the effect of psychotropic drugs as well as in **near-death** experiences where our conscious brain disappears (lower *Alpha waves*), we are capable to access and **review all our life** stored in our subconscious mind. At that moment, we are displaying brain waves like the hypnotic ones, particularly *Gamma waves* related to highly cognitive functions such as concentration, dreams, meditation, memory retrieval, conscious awareness, and those linked to memory flashbacks (attended visual stimulus). This is related with serotoninergic psychedelic chemicals (LSD or ayahuasca or endogenous **DMT- dimethyltryptamine**) influencing visual cortex. People think (not demonstrated yet) that a relevant source of endogenous DMT origin is the pineal gland, since it controls the

DOES EVIL EXIST?

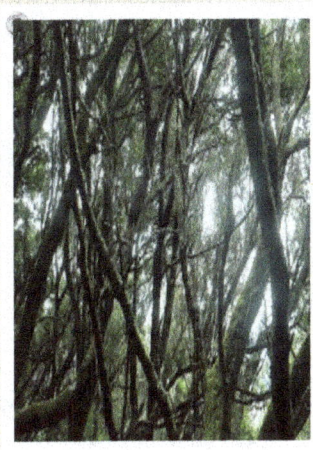

WISDOM LIFE

- If someone wants **to hurt you,**   notice the pain he hides.
- If someone wants **to lie you,**   look at the emptiness he holds.
- If someone wants **to betray you,**   notice the loneliness he carries.
- If someone **makes fun of you,**   watch the traumas he gathers.
- If someone **belittles you,**   notice how great his misery is.
- If someone **envies you,**   watch his inner frustration.

Take a good look at its flaws and try to understand them. Do not feel offended by the returns of others.

Your duty is to correct everything that prevents you from being kind and good with those who most need your help.

A WISDOM MAN ADVISE:

If someone wants **to hurt you**, notice the pain he hides.

If someone wants **to lie you**, look at the emptiness he holds.

If someone wants **to betray you**, notice the loneliness he carries.

If someone **makes fun of you**, watch the traumas he gathers.

If someone **belittles you**, notice how great his misery is.

If someone **envies you**, watch his inner frustration.

Take a good look at its flaws and try to understand them. Do not feel offended by the returns of others, your duty is to correct everything that prevents you from being kind and good with those who most need your help.

In the process of Liberation, in the process to get your Trinity, in the process to merge with the Knowledge of the Universe, you can get lost.

You create your own evil. And the Machiavellian-sadistic-narcissistic-psychopathic people are the tetrad of malignancy that we will study related with the unhealthy EGO.

Similarly, we create our own life, our own universe which can be very different from people around us. How is this so? Because the outside information entering through our senses gets modify in our body and our brain. And this modification is unique, and sometimes cannot be even comparable to your neighbours. Our brain is permanently mixing sensorial information of the world with our own hypotheses and conjectures. Even the reality coming from our eyes cannot be comparable because it is modified in the visual cortex of the brain with information coming from other regions (memory, language, sound, feelings, desires…) Any perception includes imagination, and as we will analyze in the EGO chapter, the "confirmation bias" make us to undoubtedly think in the reality that we had created.

Cultural stigmas and social norms can shape our beliefs and behaviors through a process known as CULTURAL CONDIONING. Over time, repeated exposure to cultural messages can create automatic thought patterns and habits that are stored in the brain and become unconscious. This can lead to implicit biases and shape our reactions and decisions, even if we are not aware of it. Cultural Conditioning can play a role in shaping attitudes towards sensitive or controversial topics, influencing our willingness to discuss them and potentially reinforcing cultural stigmas.

CULTURAL CONDIONING refers to the process by which an individual's behavior and beliefs are shaped by the cultural norms, values, and expectations they are exposed to throughout their life. Cultural conditioning influences a range of behaviors, including attitudes, values, beliefs, and biases. In terms of brain path, cultural conditioning can shape the development of neural circuits in the brain, including those related to decision-making and social cognition. When an individual is repeatedly exposed to cultural messages and norms, their brain forms associations between certain stimuli (such as cultural symbols or values) and the corresponding behaviors or beliefs. Over time, these associations can become automatic and ingrained in the brain, shaping the individual's perceptions, attitudes, and actions in ways that are consistent with cultural norms, even if the individual is not consciously aware of these influences. This is an ongoing process and can be influenced by a range of factors, including personal experiences, individual differences, and ongoing exposure to cultural messages.

More details regarding social conditioning can be studied in the Dopamine life chapter talking or fanaticism and in the Ego chapter.

This is the way our brain can modify the reality faced by someone, which let you to understand the difficulties to be objective building the history. And the sense of truth of audio and visual illusions under psychedelic drugs or in schizophrenia.

The observer is who build the world.

Here I enclose a personal experience in my family: *My father died when I was 12 years old. He went to the toiled and felt bad (probably an embolism) and he asked for help. I came immediately because I was in his room and helped him to arrive to the bed and asked for help to my mother that was slightly far, phoning the doctor. I was surprised when latter on, my mother explained totally convinced, that she went to help my father at the toiled and brought him to the bed. And that narrative had been stablished in the mind of my mother during all her life as a truth. I want to understand that she was guilty not to stay with him the last moment and that the only thing she remembered from that desperate situation was the story told by me and that she internalized as done by herself.*

The essential role of the observer building the world is the core of **Quantum Theory**, based on the principle of wave-particle duality, which states that particles can exhibit both wave-like and particle-like behavior depending on how they are observed. The idea is that the observer's consciousness plays a role in determining the outcome of the quantum system.

We will approach this HUMAN SUBJECTIVITY more extensively in the chapter of THE VERB.

sleep and therefore dreams. What we know is that DMT increase not only in brain but in all body under hypoxia (lack of oxygen) getting inactivated by the MAO enzyme as other Nervous System aromatic amines such as epinephrine, norepinephrine and **dopamine**.

Do you understand it? Did you like it? Every time you finish a work or get immerse in a renewal you should go to a hypnotic process to find yourself, what cares, what is your passion and your life meaning.

> Follow your purpose, in something you could create by your own.

We attract people with similar "inner values" (the ones you should discover) creating an <u>appropriate ecosystem for success</u>. Do not sacrifice yourself for your selfies, and don't confuse self-work by a network, because people with huge networks might have no self-work capable to bring them joy. Rediscover your purpose and regain your bliss. Live out of the FOMO (Fear Of Missing Out).

Never forget … YOU ARE ENOUGH, perfectly built to take care. Meaning, to reach the 4 goals in life DHARMA-KHAMA-ARTHA-MOKSHA: (1) Follow your purpose, your bliss; (2) Sensual delight through the 5 senses. Being mindful of every sense we experience, to become joyful (3) Currency (or wealth) a way we exchange our values. Our "soul profile" determine what our "inner values" are. When we exchange our inner values, we do currency (circulation) and exchanging currency is what money is. ==Therefore, you can <u>generate a lot of money</u> if you know what your values are, and you exchange with people those values (<u>no other way</u> is capable to bring wealth)==. (4) Achieve the Liberation, where the profound knowledge of yourself lets to see your mind, body, and soul directly connected and mutually influenced. We all are unique, we can't get the same type of liberation because our bodies require different ways to grow in mind, body, and soul.

I hope you enjoyed the knowledge and use it to storytelling your offprints. Our first task in education is "to shake life but leave it free to develop" and fair-tells are lies helping to understand life.

> Fight for your Self-esteem and include life acceptance and abandonment in the process.
>
> Self-esteem makes you feel fearless, independent of the good or bad opinions of the world, a winning recipe for success.

Do not translate the "law of attraction" as the majority do by "BE POSITIVE". Because it can be very stressful if you are not feeling positive, and it can exasperate others thinking you are pretending. The force comes from an **"AWAKEN MIND" open to resources such intuition or creativity.** Waking up is **about evolution**, is about acquiring higher consciousness, and reaching an infinite potential that belongs by nature to every human being. Intention *coming from the Ego* is weak, INTENTION must be born in *Your Values* the ones coming from your "soul profile" to be able to produce an invincible true success.

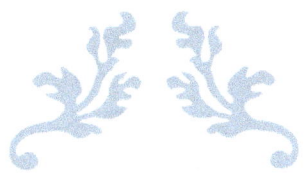

If we keep in mind that **The Soul** is the source of a **person's consciousness**, thoughts, feelings, and actions, we should face the **Theory of Mind** (cognitive theory) that determine that humans and other animals possess the ability to attribute "mental states", such as beliefs, desires, intentions, and emotions, to themselves and others. This ability is thought to be crucial for understanding the behavior of others and predicting their actions. It is an essential component of MORAL REASONING, as it allows individuals to take the perspective of others and to understand their thoughts, feelings, and intentions. This understanding is crucial for making MORAL JUDGMENTS, as it allows individuals to take into account the mental states of others when determining whether an action is right or wrong.

Keep in mind that In moral reasoning there are two views

A) Utilitarianism. Meaning to maximize collective wellbeing and happiness. Holds that moral rightness is determined by its consequences. That includes rational.
B) Deontology. There are inherent moral rules and obligations which are independent of their consequences. That includes emotions.

Several brain regions are involved in moral judgement.

➤ The ventromedial prefrontal cortex (vmPFC) is thought to play a role in evaluating the emotional value of moral dilemmas.
➤ The dorsolateral prefrontal cortex (dlPFC) is thought to play a role in cognitive control and rule-based decision making.
➤ The anterior cingulate cortex (ACC) is thought to be involved in conflict detection and resolution.
➤ The temporo-parietal junction (TPJ) is thought to be involved in understanding other people's mental states and perspective taking.
➤ The amygdala or Fear Center is thought to play a role in emotional processing and the modulation of moral judgments.
➤ Overall, these brain regions work together in a complex network to support moral judgment. Without the central node in the right temporo-parietal junction (rTPJ) we lose the mental capability to separate the consequences of an action from the intention, motivation and knowledge.

Therefore, A and B decisions are codified separately in the brain. "A decision", more rational is codified in the lateral part of the frontal cortex, the dlPFC. "B decisions", more emotional are codified in the middle part of the frontal cortex, the vmPFC.

To use the rational utilitarianism or the emotional moral rules (lateral versus medial) depends on the brain functioning at that moment. For example, using a second language the rational part is activated, while in the family or loving ones the emotional part is primarily functioning.

We create the evil.

The theory is that moral decision-making involves a balance between emotional and cognitive processes in the prefrontal cortex. Emotional processes (vmPFC), such as empathy and moral intuition, may be more strongly involved in processing MORAL GOOD, while cognitive processes (dlPFC), such as rule-based reasoning, may be more involved in processing MORAL EVIL.

Some people believe that The Soul is the source of a person's mental states and consciousness, and that it provides the basis for the Theory of Mind. Others believe that the theory of mind is a product of cognitive and neural processes, and that it does not require the existence of a soul.

Remember that all actions, intentions, knowledge, emotions get stored in the unconscious mind, this part of the mind that we can access dreaming or under hypnosis. It is our repository, and we have the ability to recall it as it happens with psychedelic drugs or in the near-death experiences (see also the Serotonin Syndrome).

> In any case, the cognitive connection between actions and its consequences is not totally achieved until the total maturation of the prefrontal cortex around the age of 25.

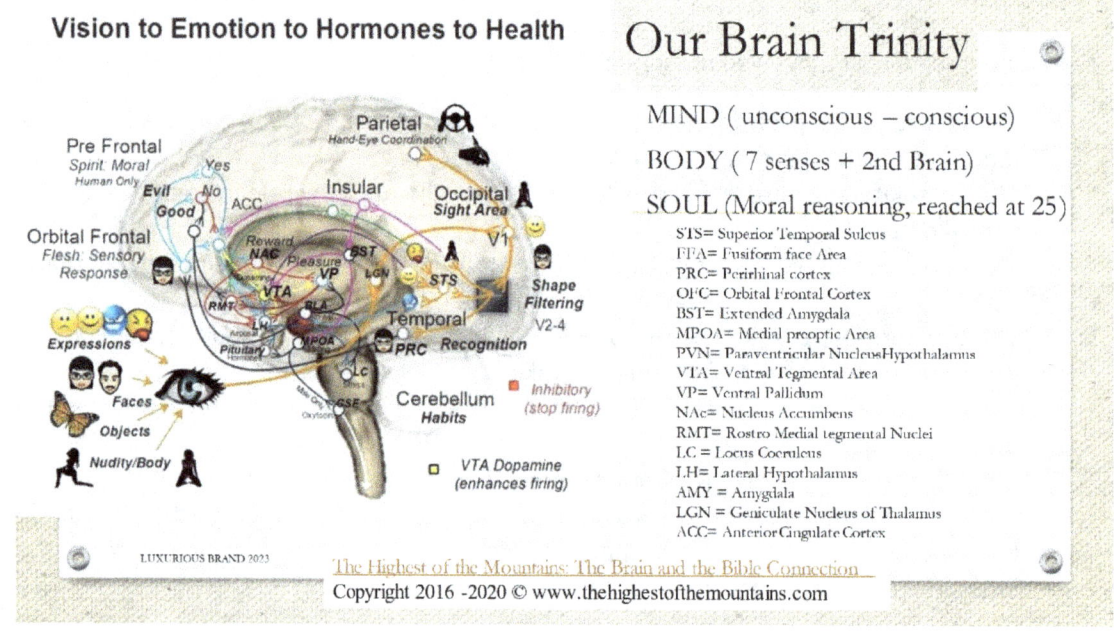

Summary of all the Brain Nuclei related with emotions, consciousness and reward.

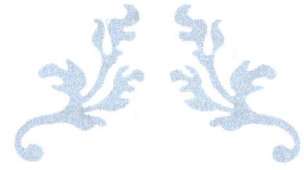

HEALING

How you create POSITIVITY and how you maintain it is the topic this time. A relevant one, the goal of Positive Psychology and the target of Coaching because **it leads to success**.
Positivity is associated to self-satisfaction, happiness, and healthiness. To reach it, you must feel good with yourself and in a healthy body capable to produce happiness hormones.

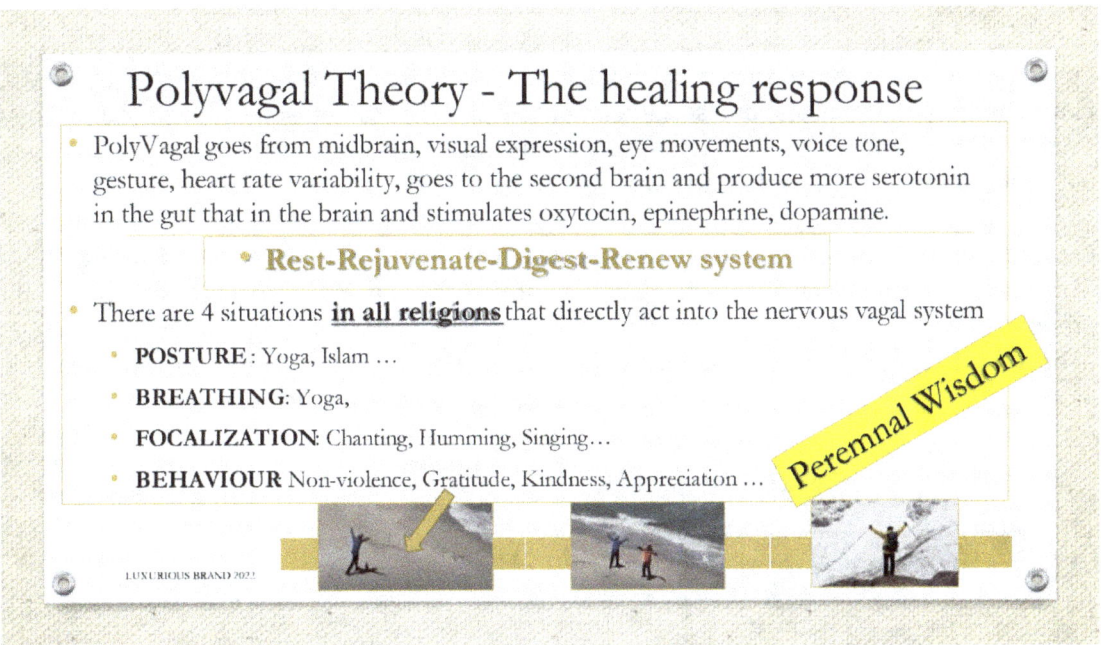

Happiness is an emotion in which interacts internal (endogenic) and external (exogenic) factors conforming the Quality of Life. Happiness hormones belong to Parasympathetic Polyvagal Healing Response the one that 'Rest- Rejuvenate- Digest & Renew'

your body **Happiness Hormones**	Mood function
Serotonin	Mood stabilizer, wellbeing, **happiness**, optimism, satisfaction. Lower down in depression. Communicates via ENS enteric nervous system of gut; able to support mental wellbeing by taking care of gut bacteria and diet.
Dopamine	**Pleasure**, motivation brain's **reward system**, positive mood. Attention, focus. Maternal behavior. 50% produced in gut.
Oxytocin	**Bonding**, love, trust, **cuddle** hormone. With pets, friendship. Counter-cortisol.
Endorphins	**Pain reliever**, runner's high, **euphoria**, bind opioid receptors, relaxation. Produced in continuous exercise, fear, love, music, chocolate eating, laughter, sex, orgasm, meditation... (endorphin +dopamine **is addictive!**)
Norepinephrine	Positively colors the emotional perception of facial expressions in humans Role in mirror neurons.
Melatonin	@brain. Circadian rhythm control by light, increase at night. Happiness and antidepressant.

Genes: Hormone release is regulated by our genes. The **Serotonin** have L=long and S=short alleles. Those receiving 2L alleles are 35% life-satisfied in front of the 19% with 2S forms. This specific gen influences serotonin, dopamine, and norepinephrine and is in **chromosome X**. Now you understand why mood and happiness of man and woman are different. Women leave with an extra-dose of those genes (loneliness affect more men while intuition is higher in women). Moreover, young women have oxytocin release every half month, during pregnancy and in lactation. On the overall, genes count 35-50% influencing happiness.

Oxytocin causes a wide spectrum of bonding behavioral being essential in maternal, sexual, family, and social. Happiness and social relationship correlates in most individuals (not all) and oxytocin provide happiness facilitating social connections. It is essential in our children and pets' relationship, and it blasts with hugs.

Predominance of brain hemispheres Left (positive) and Right (negative) also have a role. Those with Left predominance in resting phase are more positive than those with right predominance. CREATIVITY is in the RIGHT hemisphere; therefore, artists and left-handed people have tendency to negative mood. Artists could end scene performance with negative mood unless lift up with applauses/success or they have a solid and rich inner life.

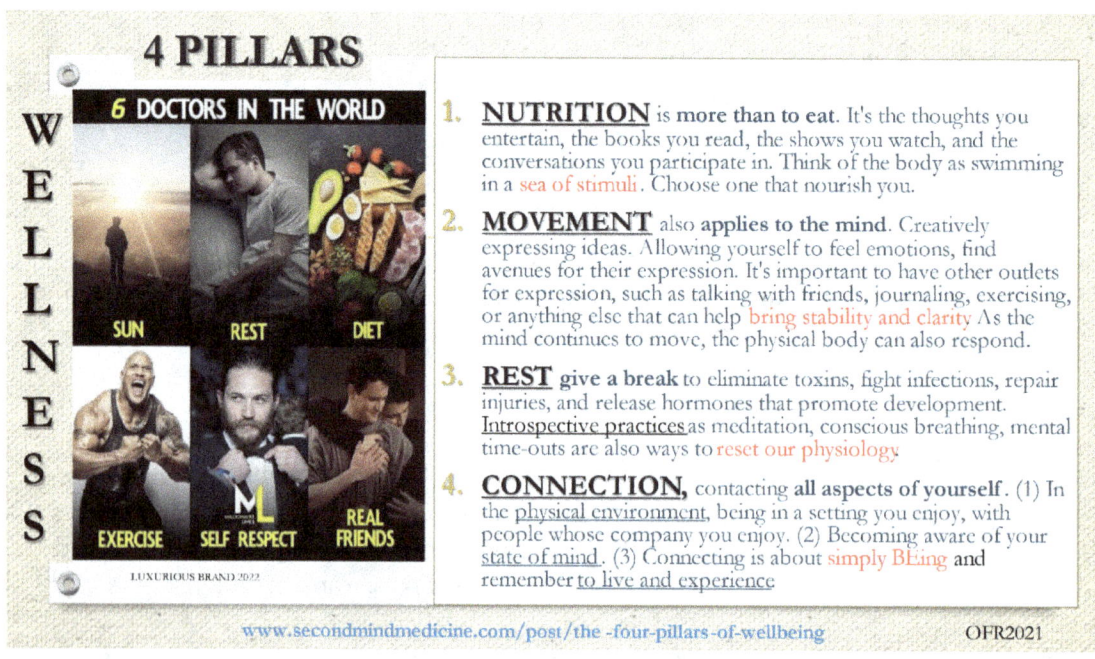

4 PILLARS

6 DOCTORS IN THE WORLD

SUN — REST — DIET

EXERCISE — SELF RESPECT — REAL FRIENDS

LUXURIOUS BRAND 2022

1. **NUTRITION** is more than to eat. It's the thoughts you entertain, the books you read, the shows you watch, and the conversations you participate in. Think of the body as swimming in a sea of stimuli. Choose one that nourish you.

2. **MOVEMENT** also **applies to the mind.** Creatively expressing ideas. Allowing yourself to feel emotions, find avenues for their expression. It's important to have other outlets for expression, such as talking with friends, journaling, exercising, or anything else that can help bring stability and clarity As the mind continues to move, the physical body can also respond.

3. **REST give a break** to eliminate toxins, fight infections, repair injuries, and release hormones that promote development. Introspective practices as meditation, conscious breathing, mental time-outs are also ways to reset our physiology

4. **CONNECTION,** contacting **all aspects of yourself.** (1) In the physical environment, being in a setting you enjoy, with people whose company you enjoy. (2) Becoming aware of your state of mind. (3) Connecting is about simply BEing and remember to live and experience

www.secondmindmedicine.com/post/the-four-pillars-of-wellbeing   OFR2021

Healthiness, there is no clear whether is healthiness who influences mood and happiness, or the opposite health is assuring our hormone well function. But what it is no doubt is that whatever the reason is, positive mood and happiness decrease the number of illnesses.

The four pillars of well-being - Nutrition, Movement, Rest, and Connection - are widely recognized as essential for a healthy and balanced life. However, these terms often have deeper implications for our mental and spiritual health that are not always fully understood.

- Nutrition is more than just what we eat. It also encompasses how we nourish our minds and spirits, such as through positive self-talk and a healthy relationship with food.
- Movement goes beyond physical exercise and also refers to mental and emotional movement, such as exploring new experiences and perspectives.

- Rest is not limited to simply sleeping. It includes taking breaks from stressors, engaging in self-care, and finding time for reflection and relaxation.
- Connection is not only about socializing with others, but also about connecting with ourselves, nature, and our higher purpose.

By recognizing the full scope of these four pillars, we can strive for a more holistic and well-rounded approach to wellness and well-being.

Many exceptions will be cover in other chapters, particularly in the role of our Neurotransmitters, but REST required special attention since it influences at least seven aspects as can be seen in the next image of the Sacred Rest.

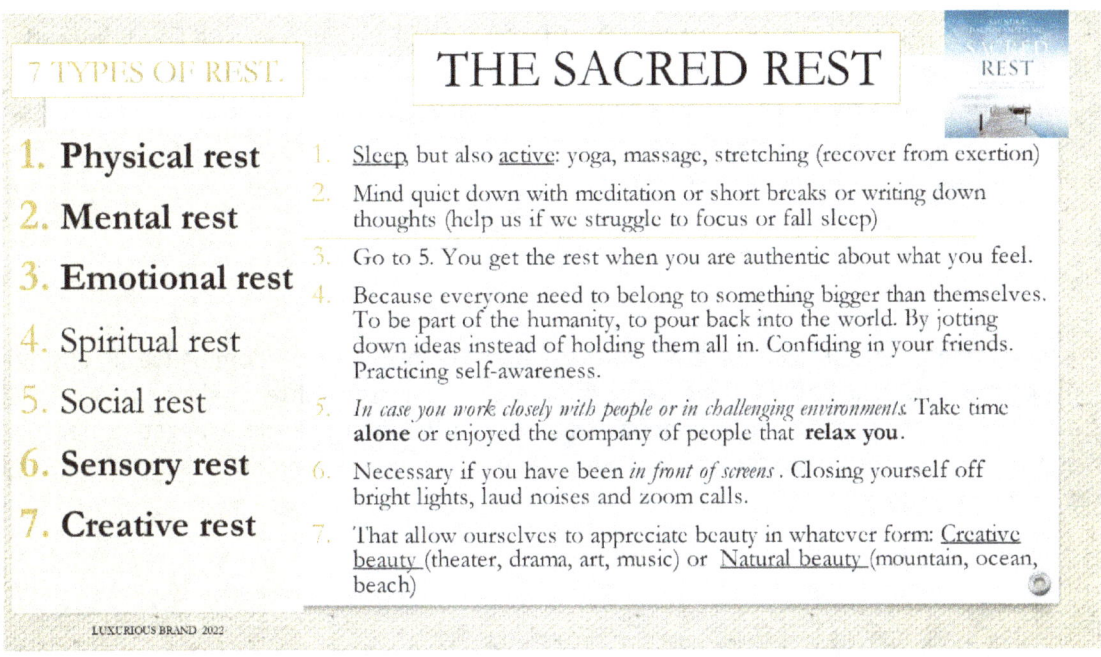

Apart from the five more obvious types of rest that contribute to overall well-being such as:

1. Physical rest: This includes sleeping and taking breaks from physical activity to allow the body to recover and recharge.
2. Mental rest: This involves taking breaks from mentally taxing activities, such as work or school, and engaging in leisure activities or mindfulness practices.
3. Emotional rest: This includes taking breaks from emotional stressors and practicing self-care activities to reduce stress and improve emotional well-being.
4. Spiritual rest: This involves connecting with one's sense of purpose and taking time for reflection, meditation, and other spiritual practices.
5. Social rest: This involves taking breaks from social interactions and giving yourself time and space to recharge.

There are another two recently included: **Sensory rest,** as a result of persistent exposure to the blue light of screens, laud music and teleworking. **Creative rest**, by engaging in creative activities, individuals can tap into their sense of wonder and appreciate the beauty in their surroundings. This can help to foster a deeper connection with the world and improve overall well-being. Examples of creative activities that can be used to appreciate beauty include Photography, Painting or drawing, Music, Poetry or creative writing, Gardening...

Self-respect, the opinion of ourselves including our outside body do directly affect our mood and happiness. Similarly, attractive people are perceived as happier and successful. When people are considered attractive, we associate that they are more intelligent, kindly and with more social skills (the "Halo Effect" that can be studied in The Ego chapter). Bias to attractiveness is easily traceable, and attractive people must cope with it, assume it and **use it for good**, in their social influence. Nevertheless, **attractiveness** is enriched by an inside effect that reflect our own opinions and the richness of our inner life, and sometimes its strong perception could overpass the aspect of our physical body (i.e. Mother Therese of Calcutta).

Stress: Cortisol (depression and anxiety-neuroticism) and **Adrenaline** do not belong to the happiness hormones; they are Stress Hormones (fight-or-flight response of the Sympathetic nervous system). Slightly, it could be helpful to focus outside of you, releasing Endorphins. But too much is destructive, depress immunological system, burn us out, destroying the capability of recovery (except for "high altruistic reasons" but never should be persistent too long on time). Individuals with higher levels of "personal growth" and "purpose in life" have lower and more stable levels of Cortisol and Adrenaline.

POSITIVITY

We mentioned the influence of the Right-Left brain hemisphere predominance in positive feelings and how genes or healthiness also intervenes. Neurotransmitters balance that we will study in following chapters are essential. But noticed, women are more negative because negative feelings are associated to take care of the offspring, demanding to be aware at any risk that could appear.

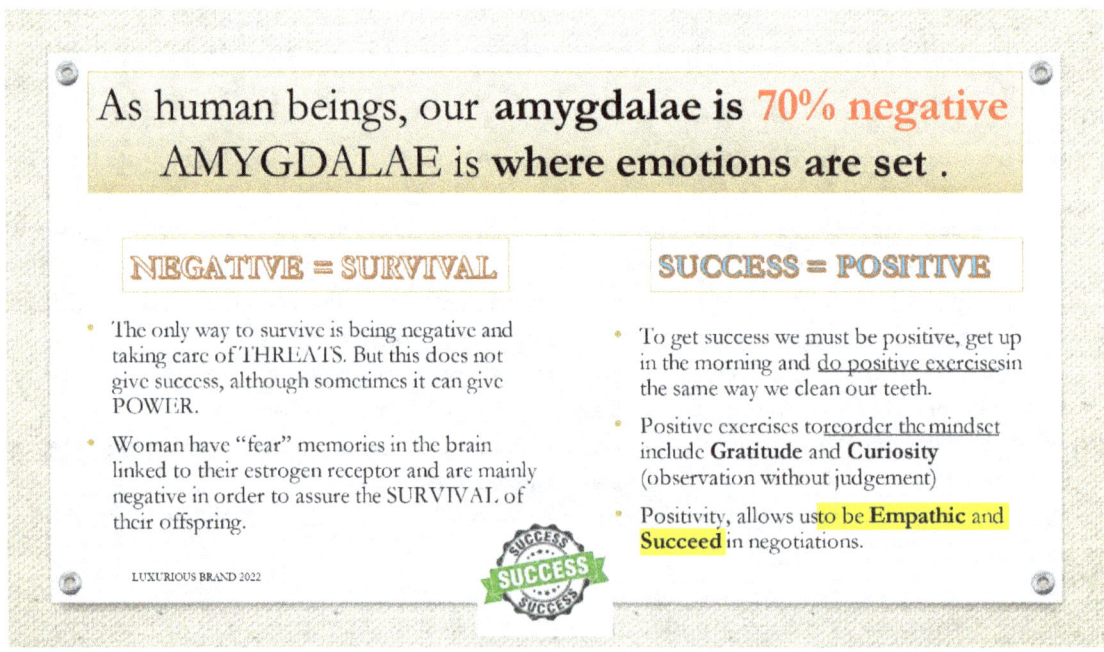

As human beings, our **amygdalae is 70% negative** AMYGDALAE is **where emotions are set** .

NEGATIVE = SURVIVAL

- The only way to survive is being negative and taking care of THREATS. But this does not give success, although sometimes it can give POWER.
- Woman have "fear" memories in the brain linked to their estrogen receptor and are mainly negative in order to assure the SURVIVAL of their offspring.

LUXURIOUS BRAND 2022

SUCCESS = POSITIVE

- To get success we must be positive, get up in the morning and do positive exercises in the same way we clean our teeth.
- Positive exercises to reorder the mindset include **Gratitude** and **Curiosity** (observation without judgement)
- Positivity, allows us to be **Empathic** and **Succeed** in negotiations.

The amygdala is involved in processing emotions, although not for setting all of our emotions. Its major role is processing FEAR and other negative emotions with a clear goal: *"To survive we must be negative in order to take care of Threats"*. The amygdala or FEAR CENTER have two tasks 1) Scan the environment for threats and 2) Talk with the rest of the brain to handle them. The amygdala is our emotional processor and our moral judgments modulator, but those are exclusively evaluated on the premises of Fear to Threats.

To survive you must show POWER, in other words show the **HARM** you could produce, an expression of a **negative perception**, fact that we will develop later in the EGO's chapter and people's vibrations.

But to get **SUCCESS** we must be positive, we must develop Empathy and Trust, in other words we must fight against our negative primitive amygdala using our Prefrontal Cortex (PFC) the executive function of our CONSCIOUS brain.

The response of our primitive amygdala is to activate the hypothalamic-pituitary-adrenal (HPA) axis. In other words, to activate our response to Stress, the fight-or-flight response of our Sympathetic nervous system. A good level of stress is determinant of our motivation releasing Dopamine due to the amygdala connection with the VTA (*Ventral Tegmental Area*). But a bad level of stress is determinant of a Chronic Stress consuming our hormonal resources, downregulating neurotransmitters receptors (by overexcitation) inducing tolerance and ending into cell death (by excitotoxicity) and depression. And remember when neurons died, they not come back and when receptors disappear, they require 1 year to come back.

Furthermore, the amygdala is always in reciprocity connection with the *Hippocampus,* which is the Memory Center of the brain, where our memory resides, and where all those Threats and Fears will be stored.

Everyone has both positive and negative thoughts and behaviors, but not everyone is aware that these negative thoughts will persist unless not actively addressed, transforming the statement "Don't worry, be happy" into an essential one. The reason for this peculiar fact is that our active brain is not able to subtract or divide memories (in this case negative thoughts).

==Our active brain can only sum up or multiply.==

Therefore, it's not advisable to simply ask or pray for negative thoughts to disappear, as they will only become stronger. Instead, you should take proactive steps to forget these thoughts. The process of "pruning" in the brain, where non-essential memories are trimmed away, only occurs when a memory is not frequently accessed or deemed unimportant. So, by not constantly focusing on negative thoughts, they may eventually fade away naturally. Additionally, during sleep, the brain is able to further prune away memories that are not frequently used.

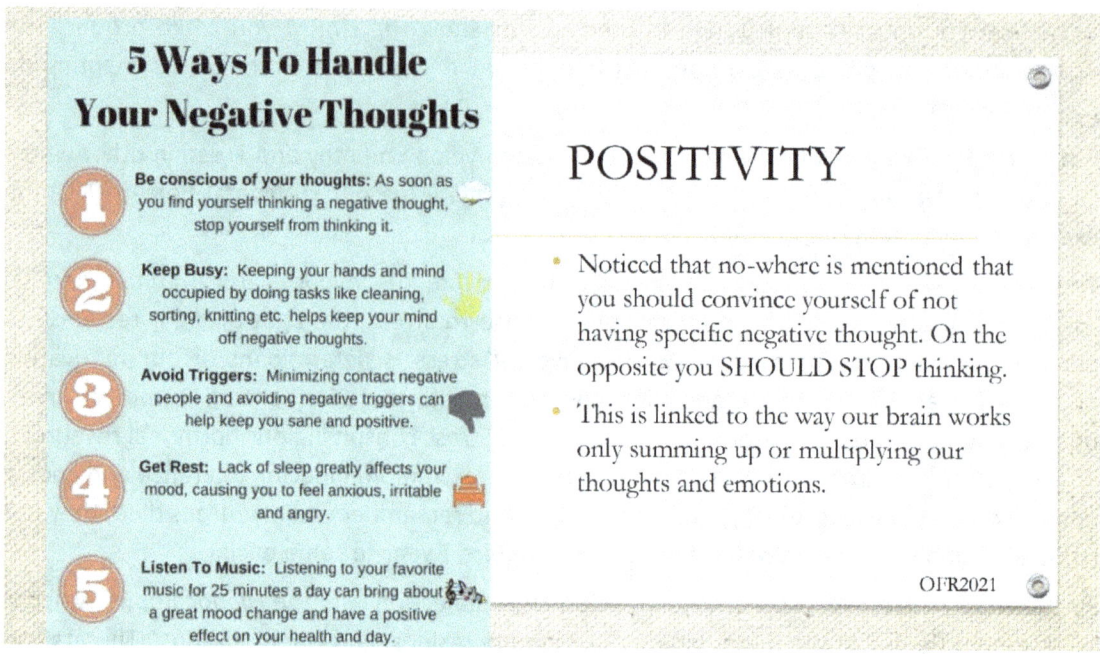

5 Ways To Handle Your Negative Thoughts

1. **Be conscious of your thoughts:** As soon as you find yourself thinking a negative thought, stop yourself from thinking it.

2. **Keep Busy:** Keeping your hands and mind occupied by doing tasks like cleaning, sorting, knitting etc. helps keep your mind off negative thoughts.

3. **Avoid Triggers:** Minimizing contact negative people and avoiding negative triggers can help keep you sane and positive.

4. **Get Rest:** Lack of sleep greatly affects your mood, causing you to feel anxious, irritable and angry.

5. **Listen To Music:** Listening to your favorite music for 25 minutes a day can bring about a great mood change and have a positive effect on your health and day.

POSITIVITY

- Noticed that no-where is mentioned that you should convince yourself of not having specific negative thought. On the opposite you SHOULD STOP thinking.

- This is linked to the way our brain works only summing up or multiplying our thoughts and emotions.

OFR2021

Here are several ways to cultivate positive thoughts:

1. Practice gratitude: Make a habit of focusing on what you are thankful for in your life.
2. Surround yourself with positive people: Seek out relationships with individuals who have a positive outlook and support your goals.
3. Engage in activities you enjoy: Do things that bring you joy and fulfillment.
4. Focus on the present moment: Mindfulness practices can help you stay focused on the present and avoid getting caught up in negative thoughts about the past or future.
5. Set achievable goals: Accomplishing even small goals can boost self-esteem and provide a sense of accomplishment.
6. Practice self-care: Take care of your physical, emotional, and mental well-being.
7. Seek out humor: Laughing and smiling can release feel-good chemicals in the brain and help you to feel more positive.
8. Focus on the positive: Try to notice and focus on positive things in your life, rather than dwelling on negatives.

And the next image showed how the humps holding memories are seen in the neuron prolongations, those that will be pruned during sleep if they are not frequently used.

HOW WE ELIMINATE MEMORIES

SLEEP REM PHASE

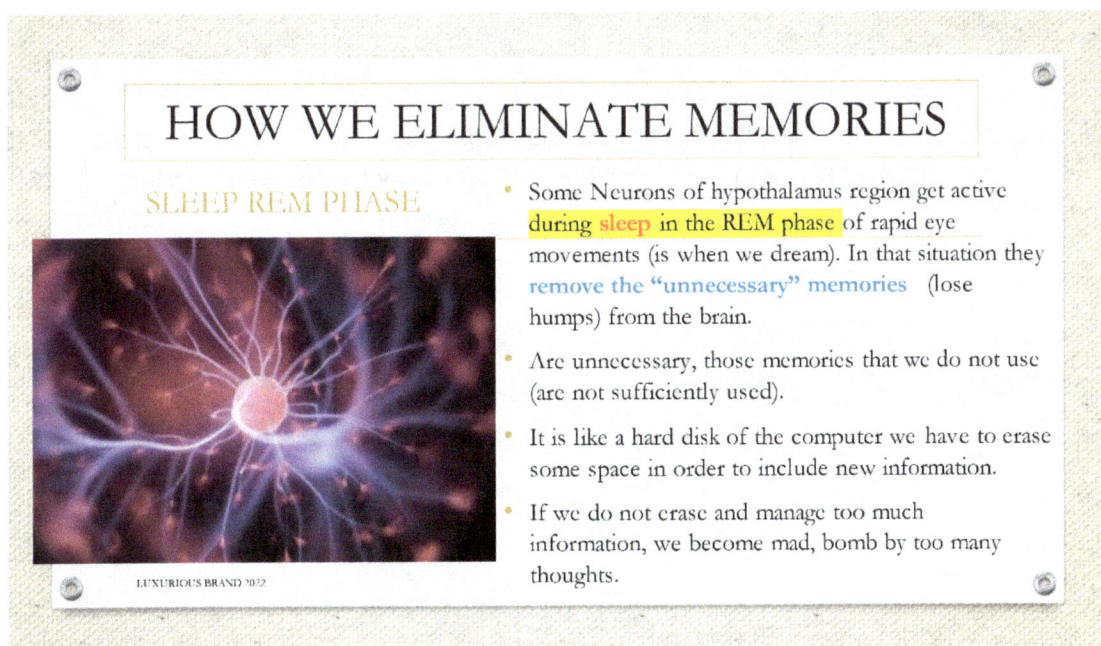

LUXURIOUS BRAND 2022

- Some Neurons of hypothalamus region get active during sleep in the REM phase of rapid eye movements (is when we dream). In that situation they remove the "unnecessary" memories (lose humps) from the brain.

- Are unnecessary, those memories that we do not use (are not sufficiently used).

- It is like a hard disk of the computer we have to erase some space in order to include new information.

- If we do not erase and manage too much information, we become mad, bomb by too many thoughts.

The conclusion is very easy: concentrate in other things to evanish humps with negative thoughts in order to assure not to make them bigger.

In other words: "Don't worry, be happy."

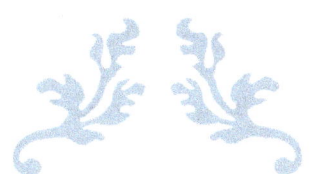

MULTILAYERED BODY

Clairvoyance, clairsentience, clair cognizance, clairaudience, synesthesia ... it is obvious that there are a lot of perspectives in our bodies that are not widely recognized because our body is in fact multilayered.

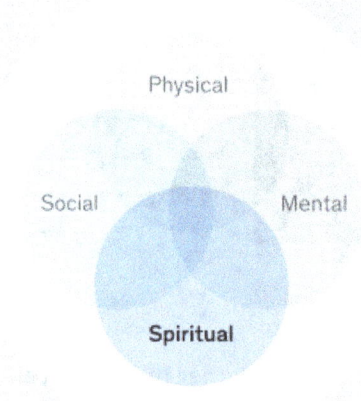

- Physical Body = Physician-Homeopath
- Spiritual Body = ENERGY (blockages)
- Emotional Body = HEART (origin)
- Mental Body = BELIEFS- REASONING

To face an inclusive medicine, we not only have to refer the body as a physical body, but we must recognize that is much more than this. And that the core or the center of this is the INFINITE CONSCIOUSNESS, the totipotential consciousness (identified or related to God, to the Creator).

To recognize this, we should know first ourselves including not only our body but our mind.

DEFAULT MODE NETWORK

It starts in recognizing and potentiate our brain **Default Mode Network (DMN)** the most active part of the brain when an individual is not focused on the outside world, but in **our inside body** (our consciousness) such as when they are daydreaming, mind-wandering, or recalling events from their past. It has been referred to as the **"me center"** of the brain because it is involved in self-referential processing, such as thinking about one's own thoughts, feelings, and experiences. The DMN is thought to play an important role in the integration of information from different brain regions and in the creation of a coherent sense of self. DMN regulates our memory and internal thoughts, and it is known to be vulnerable to stress-like-toxicity, aging and disease.

Some of the key integrators of the DMN include:

1. Medial Prefrontal Cortex (mPFC): This region is involved in self-referential processing and decision-making.

2. Posterior Cingulate Cortex (PCC): This region is involved in the processing of autobiographical memories and self-referential thoughts.
3. Hippocampus: This region is involved in the formation and retrieval of long-term memories and is important for episodic memory.
4. Temporoparietal Junction (TPJ): This region is involved in perspective-taking and empathy and is thought to play a role in the integration of information from different sources.
5. Retrosplenial Cortex: Situated in the posterior part of the cingulate cortex and adjacent to the precuneus, involved in memory integration, spatial navigation, and creating a sense of space.
6. Anterior Precuneus (aPCu): Located in the precuneus, it is an important component of the DMN involved in establishing our physical self, integrating spatial information, sensory input, and proprioceptive signals to contribute to our self-awareness and sense of body ownership.

Furthermore, the brain is integrated by multiple, interacting networks that support different functions and behaviors. Some of those networks are:

- Task Positive Network (TPN): This network is active when an individual is focused on a specific task and it is involved in attention and executive functions.
- Salience Network: This network helps to allocate attention to important stimuli and is involved in switching between different mode networks.
- Sensorimotor Network: This network is involved in processing sensory information from the body and coordinating movement.
- Visual Network: This network is involved in processing visual information and is active during tasks that require visual attention.
- Default Mode Network (DMN) as we explain in charge of the coherent sense of self.

Relationship between brain waves and specific mental states or cognitive processes is complex as we have referred extensively in the hypnosis chapter. But when our brain is in the Default Mode the alpha rhythm is the predominant. **Alpha waves** are characterized by a frequency of 8-12 Hz and are most prominent in the posterior regions of the brain, such as the temporoparietal junction and the posterior cingulate cortex. Alpha activity is thought to reflect a state of idleness or low arousal and is often associated with a lack of external stimulation, meaning that we are self-centered with a low-level background activity characteristic of the DMN. Conversely, when the DMN is suppressed, such as during a task-oriented cognitive state, alpha waves are suppressed and other patterns of brain activity, such as beta or gamma waves, become more prominent.

The number of functions associated to DMN include:

- Memory formation and recall: The hippocampus, a key component of the DMN, is known to play a critical role in memory formation and recall.
- Self-referential thinking: The DMN is active when people reflect on their own thoughts, emotions, and experiences.
- Social cognition: The DMN is also involved in processing social and emotional information, allowing individuals to understand the thoughts and feelings of others.
- Mental health: Abnormal activity in the DMN has been associated with various mental health conditions, including depression, anxiety, and schizophrenia.

Recent studies have linked exposure to environmental pollution, particularly air pollution, with changes in brain function, including alterations in the activity of the DMN that loose connectivity which reduce cognitive abilities and get symptoms of depression.

MULTILAYER HEALING

HEALING means RE-INTEGRATION → RESTORING INTEGRATION (if it is a cut healing restores skin continuity). To restore (heal) we must have something DISINTEGRATED.

It is obvious that we go to a doctor to heal our physical body, but <mark>HUMAN BEINGS are more than physical bodies</mark>. And we often forget to heal the rest of the layers from which HUMANS are composed.

We need a **MULTILAYER HEALING.**

We are considered integrated by at least for 5 bodies as a Human BEINGs (permanently BEING created):

1. **- CONCIOUSNESS (Fundamental Flow-Potential pool of Uncertainty)**

2. - INFORMATIONAL (in form, is passing the consciousness into the level of energy, is the notion of reality in formation, potential state of uncertainty, INFORMATION= use to remove the uncertainty)

3. - ENERGETIC (pragma, chi, chacras, vital force, chemical energy (ATP), measurable, non-measurable, kinetic, molecular vibration…)

4. - MENTAL (feelings, thoughts, intuition, …)

5. - PHYSICAL BODY (from anatomy to microscopic organelles and molecules)

#1- CONCIOUSNESS totipotential derived from the INFINITE CONCIOUSNESS.

#2-3-4 collect Experiences, it is what we **personally** are, it is a phenomenological approach.

#5 is analytical, we can measure, it is what we **physically** are.

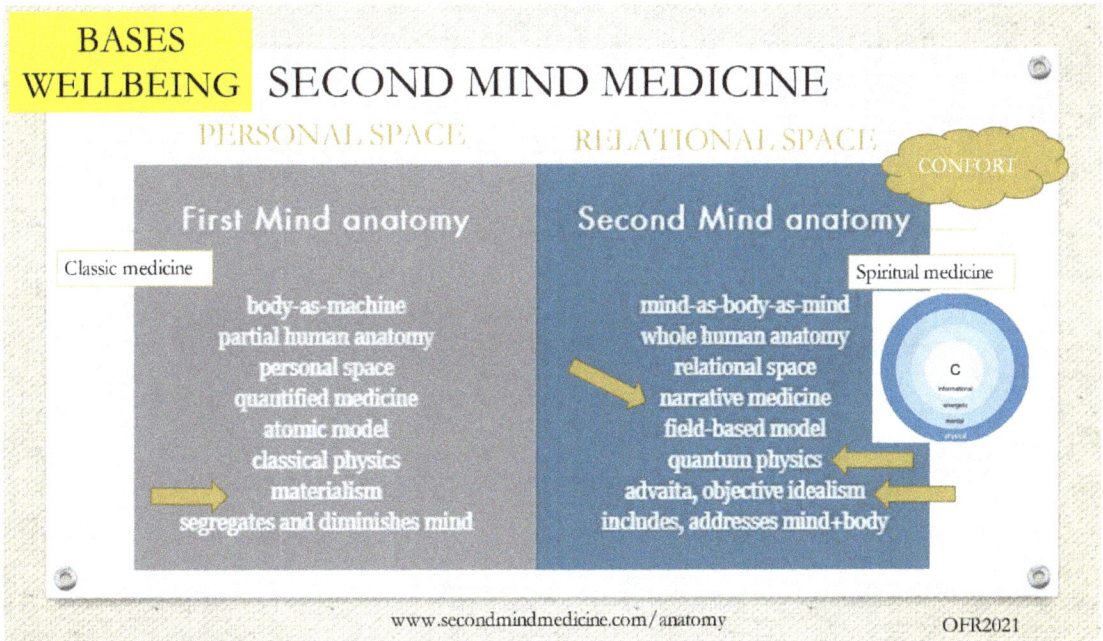

THE CONCIOUSNESS #1. The TOTIPOTENTIAL EXPERIENCE not yet concretized (interesting enough storytelling – as we will see in the chapter of the VERB- may concretize it)

THE INFORMATION #2. In charge to inform what the consciousness had concretized (could be through a storytelling). IN-FORMING to our ENERGETIC BODY#3 about our change of consciousness. Is the BRIDGE trying to form **our #3 ENERGETIC body**. A bridge between the totipotential consciousness and the first EXPERIENCE able to be detected by our owns.

    Directly affect our ENERGETIC body (concentration, no concentration, change aura…)

THE ENERGETIC BODY #3, it is directly affected by **EMOTIONS.** It is directly affected by the influence in our consciousness#1 through the information#2 → meaning that it has some healing (reintegration) or disease (disintegration) effect in our energetic body.

        Directly affects MENTAL body (fear, joy, happiness, hate, peace…)

THE MENTAL BODY #4, It is directly affected by **EMOTIONS.** It is directly affected by the ENERGETIC#3 body → meaning that it has a healing (reintegration) or disease (disintegration) effect in our mental body.

        Directly affects PHYSICAL body (tachycardia, trembling, hair erection…)

THE PHYSICAL BODY #5. It is influenced by the mental #4 and the energetic body #3 → meaning that it has a healing (reintegration) or disease (disintegration) effect in our physical body.

        Directly produce PHYSICAL effects (tachycardia, headache, cry, smile, alter respiratory rhythm…)

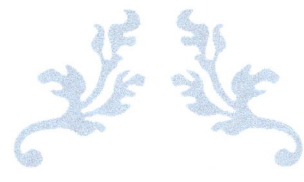

THE CASCADE OF CONSCIOUSNESS

This view is totally in coincidence of the most updated philosophical opinion of what is life and a living BEING from Humberto Maturana. Every LIVING BEING is a closed system that is CONTINUALLY CREATING ITSELF, **repairing**, maintaining, modifying, de novo creating. A cascade of life from the totipotential consciousness, since ...

> The production of ourselves constitutes the living.

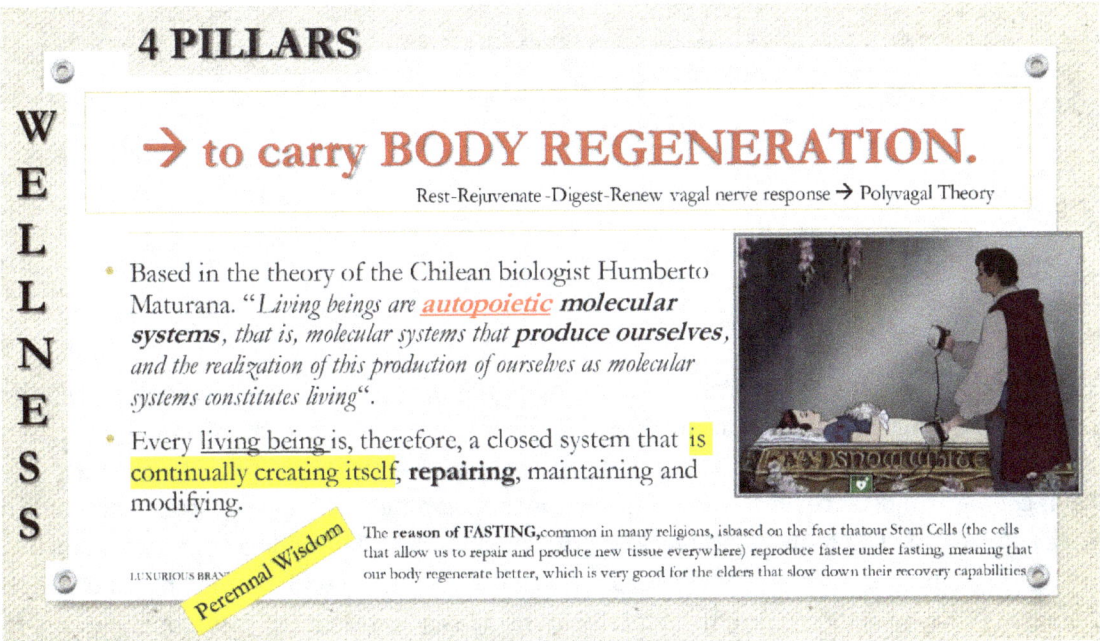

With this concept of life, some consider that the Universe is a living being, a closed system that self-perpetuates. The cosmos may possess an innate capacity to learn, adapt, and evolve in a similar way to a living organism (The Autodidactic Universe. Alexander S. et al 2021; https://arxiv.org/abs/2104.03902).

The "CASCADE OF CONCIOUSNESS" refers to the process by which living beings create and maintain their own existence, according to Humberto Maturana's philosophy of life. It is a holistic view that sees all aspects of a living organism as interconnected and interdependent and views the creation and maintenance of life as an ongoing process. In this view, consciousness plays a key role in the cascade, as it allows the organism to perceive, respond, and modify its environment in order to sustain itself, it behaves as God. The cascade of consciousness is therefore a continuous feedback loop of perception, response, and modification that allows living beings to maintain and modify their existence.

We are THE CREATORS; God is inside us.

In our physical body life depends on complex chemical compounds synthesized following genes codes, and most of our gene's regions are not active now-a-days. Furthermore, the synthesized proteins are 3D entities which life function rely upon a specific three-dimensional structure. But surprisal enough we produce an important number of intrinsically disordered proteins (IDP) or intrinsically disordered protein regions (IDPR) and each have a collection of thousands of possible distinct shapes, or ensemble. Our capabilities to create are endless.

In a most pragmatic aspect, in the following chapters we will show that we are what our neurotransmitters (an ordered type of 3D proteins) let us to be, shaping our Mental body and becoming an essential part of our healthiness, equal or more important that the one related with our physical body.

Let's make the mental health a priority.

NEUROTRANSMITERS

The **consciousness of self** is in the nervous system. Neurons transmit information through the process of synaptic transmission. In this process, a nerve impulse (action potential) travels along the axon of a neuron and triggers the release of **neurotransmitters** (3D proteins- the key), chemical substances that can cross the synaptic gap between two neurons and bind to specific receptors (3D proteins- the lock) on the next neuron. This binding triggers a change in the electrical properties of the next neuron, which leads to the initiation or inhibition of a new nerve impulse (electrical current), thereby transmitting information from one neuron to another.

The most used neurotransmitter is acetylcholine (ACh), which is involved in functions such as muscle contraction, learning, and memory. It is also involved in the regulation of heart rate and the activity of the sympathetic and parasympathetic nervous systems. Other important neurotransmitters include dopamine, serotonin, norepinephrine, GABA, and glutamate. The specific neurotransmitter and the effects it has on the body vary depending on the type of neuron and it specific function.

In this chapter we are going to understand that our fulfillment depends on neurotransmitters balance i.e imbalances in dopamine and serotonin levels can contribute to various neurological and psychiatric disorders, including depression, anxiety, and Parkinson's disease.

And that giving away neurotransmitters as a gift not only make us happy but create happiness in our surroundings.

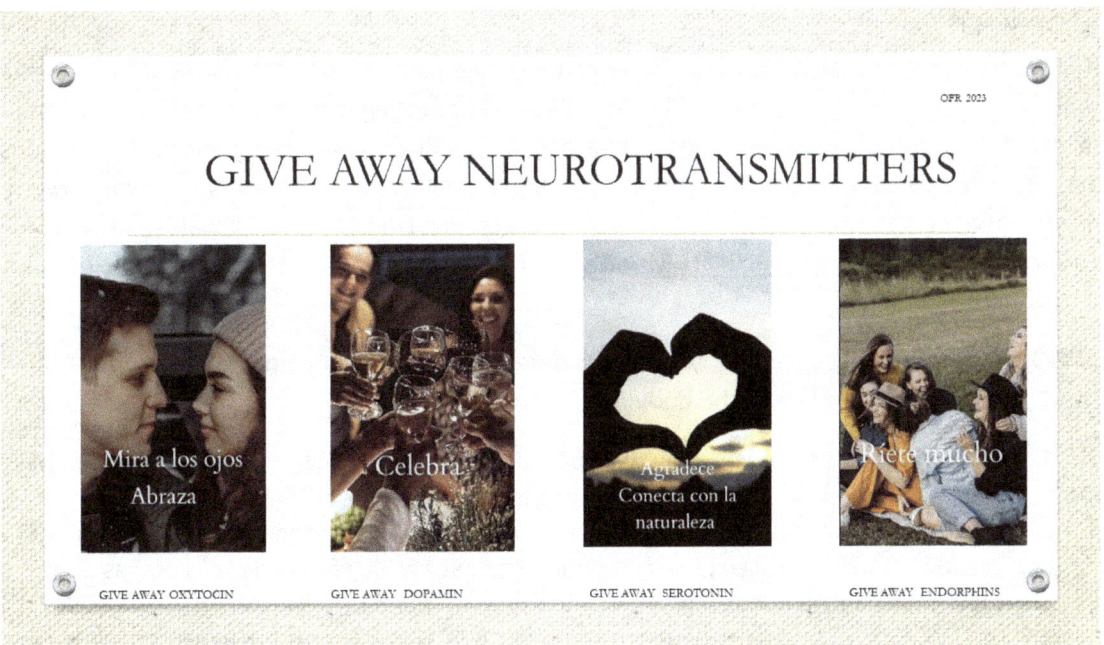

==We are what our neurotransmitters let us to be.==

Maybe you are first curious to know how scientists have found links between neurotransmitters and behavior. The research methods usually used are:

- Animal Studies: Scientists can manipulate the levels of neurotransmitters in animals and observe the effect on behavior.
- Brain Imaging Studies: Advances in brain imaging technology have allowed scientists to visualize the activity of neurotransmitters in the human brain and see how it relates to behavior. For example, PET (positron emission tomography) scans can show the distribution of neurotransmitter receptors in the brain, while fMRI (functional magnetic resonance imaging) can show changes in brain activity in response to different stimuli.
- Clinical Trials: Clinical trials with human subjects can provide more direct evidence of the relationship between neurotransmitters and behavior. For example, trials can test the effect of drugs that target specific neurotransmitters, such as antidepressants that increase serotonin levels, on behavior.
- Observational Studies: Observational studies can identify correlations between neurotransmitter levels and behavior in human subjects. For example, studies have found a correlation between low levels of serotonin and depression, and between high levels of dopamine and increased risk-taking behavior.

A neurotransmitter may be linked to a particular behavior, but it is likely that other factors, such as genetics, environment, and other brain processes, also play a role.

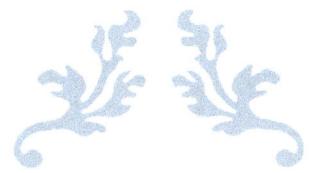

ENDORPHIN

It is worth to know that with hypnosis we can produce pain relieve at the level of anesthesia thanks to our neurotransmitters. This is achieved activating certain regions of the brain involved in pain perception and modulating neurotransmitters of pain signaling. Pain regions according to functional magnetic resonance imaging (fMRI) are the *anterior cingulate cortex*, *insula*, and *dorsal rostral pons*. Neurotransmitters involved in pain signaling are mainly endorphins, our **natural PAINKILLERS** as well as Dopamine and Serotonin reducing pain perception.

ENDORPHIN is not only a painkiller, it also promotes feelings of wellbeing. There are several ways to increase endorphins in the body:

1. Exercise: Regular physical activity, especially moderate to high-intensity exercises, has been shown to increase endorphin levels and improve mood.
2. Laugh: Laughing can stimulate the release of endorphins and reduce pain perception.
3. Eat spicy foods: Capsaicin, the compound that gives spicy foods their heat, has been shown to increase endorphin levels and improve mood.
4. Get a massage: Massages have been shown to increase endorphin levels and reduce pain perception.
5. Practice mindfulness: Meditation, yoga, and other mindfulness practices have been shown to increase endorphin levels and reduce stress and anxiety.

Beta-endorphins, enkephalins, dynorphins, and their G-protein link brain opioid receptor and non-opioid receptor such nociceptin (NOP). These peptides and their receptors in *central limbic* and *paralimbic* regions are involved in the modulation of affective states, neuroendocrine and autonomic stress responses, and mood and motivational processes as well as pain.

Its effect explains why when we are loved or kissed, our pain decreases or disappears -very effective in children-. It is also the reason why the level of pain differs from one to another, and the benefits that kindness and caress have on ill people.

Endorphins are produced in response to various stimuli, including physical touch, affection, and emotional connection. Physical touch, such as a hug or kiss, triggers the release of endorphins in the body, which can help to reduce feelings of pain and discomfort. The release of endorphins is associated with increased feelings of happiness, pleasure, and well-being, which can help to distract the brain from focusing on physical pain.

In addition to the release of endorphins, emotional connection and affection can also play a role in reducing pain. When we feel loved and supported by others, it can help to reduce stress and anxiety, which can in turn decrease the perception of pain. Love and affection can also promote a sense of comfort and safety, which can help to relieve pain and discomfort.

Overall, the combination of physical touch and emotional connection can help to reduce pain and increase feelings of comfort and well-being.

DMT- Dimethyltryptamine is a chemical with a strong psychotropic effect that is naturally produced in human body, which exact location in the brain is not well understood. The neurotransmitter serotonin, involved in regulating mood, appetite, and sleep, is believed to play a role in the production and release of DMT in the brain. it is worth mention their participation in the Pineal gland, the one that allow us to fall sleep, controlling our dreams particularly at awakening. Studies have suggested that DMT may be involved in the regulation of wakefulness and dream states, as well as the regulation of mystical and spiritual experiences.

The psychotropic effect of DMT is such that carry the disappearance of conscious mind, liberating the unconscious mind that could allow us to review all our life. At that moment, we are displaying brain waves like the hypnotic ones, particularly **Gamma waves** related to highly cognitive functions such as concentration, dreams, meditation, memory retrieval, conscious awareness, and those linked to **memory flashbacks** (attended visual stimulus). Gamma waves are high-frequency brain waves involved in conscious perception and cognitive processing. Under DMT, gamma waves increase particularly in the visual cortex, contributing to the intense visual hallucinations and altered perceptions commonly reported.

DMT interacts with the brain's **SEROTONIN SYSTEM** (see in serotonin life chapter), leading to the changes in brain waves and perception, thought, and emotion by changing brain's electrical activity. It increases **alpha and theta waves** associated with altered states of consciousness, including relaxation and meditation.

Some theories suggest that DMT may be produced and released during certain stages of sleep, during near-death experiences, or during periods of intense stress or physical exertion and that could be released by any tissue in the body under high hypoxia.

But DMT is also found in various plant species, including *Psychotria viridis* and *Diplopterys cabrerana*, which are native to South America. It is also present in the bark and leaves of certain species of Acacia, which are found in Australia. And in the parotid gland of the bufo toad or *Incilius Alvarius* living in the state of Colorado-EEUU, containing 5-MeO-DMT together with Bufotenin derived from serotonin. DMT is an essential part of the **Ayahuasca** used in traditional South American shamanic rituals.

Ayahuasca is integrated by two plants only one containing DMT (a brush -*Psychotria viridi-*) and the other IMAO (the liana -*Bannisteriosis caapri-*) which is the inhibitor of monoamine oxidase. In the ritual, the disbalance of neurotransmitters produced by DMT will not be controlled by the MAO, as it should be, because it is inhibited by IMAO. When ingested, it produces intense, short-lived hallucinations, profound alterations in thought, perception, and mood, and a sense of connection to a spiritual realm. In fact, people coming from those experiences see themselves as belonging to God, assisting to a LIBERATION where our TRINITY of Mind-Body-Soul is one with the surrounding world.

The mechanism by which DMT produces its psychotropic effects is by interacting with the serotonin system in the brain. The hallucinations are very vivid and are recognized as a ***Visions***, constructions of the imagination with high visual impact. The normal route of Perceptions in the brain goes from eye.signals-thalamus-visual.cortex-memories-frontal.cortex. In ***Psychedelic Perceptions*** the route is inverted. In this case, perceptions are created internally starting in the frontal cortex and follow the inverse route frontal.cortex-memories-visual.cortex. This means that DMT is projecting our own memories into the visual cortex. In other words, DMT is presenting visually our Soul, we are able to see our Soul. Under these circumstances visual flashbacks can cover not only all our unconscious collected memories (as in the near-death experiences) but can visually connect with our origin, with our Infinite Consciousness, with God.

We must remind that DMT is a prohibited psychedelic drug due to the strong risks for life and mind in those astral trips if they are not highly supervised and controlled by experienced people.

DMT helps to distinguish our Trinity (Mind-Body-Soul) and our communion with God.

Not only DMT is prohibited, also the Psilocybin a naturally occurring psychoactive compound found in certain species of mushrooms that also release Serotonin in the brain is also prohibited for the risks of the SEROTONIN SYNDROME that we will study in the Serotonin chapter.

The effects of PSILOCYBIN can vary depending on factors such as dose, the person's state of mind and environment, and the species of mushroom from which the psilocybin was obtained. It produces Astral trips with a wide sensory experience:

- Altered perceptions of time and space
- Intensified and altered sensory experiences.
- Changes in thought patterns and a sense of increased creativity
- Mood changes, including euphoria, anxiety, and confusion.
- Spiritual or mystical experiences
- Hallucinations and altered visual and auditory perceptions.

It is important to note that the effects of psilocybin can be unpredictable, and in some cases, can be intense and unpleasant.

GLUTAMATE

Those particularly interested in learning, the **GLUTAMATE** is the main <mark>EXCITATORY neurotransmitter</mark> in the brain, involved in processes such as learning, memory, and the regulation of synaptic plasticity, regulation of muscle tone, and control of hunger. It is important in regulating mood and anxiety. It is found throughout the brain but is particularly abundant in the *cortex* and *hippocampus*.

The level of Glutamate gets reduced in stroke and epilepsy. In **stroke**, due to cell death and brain-blood barrier damage that increase **excitotoxicity**, a process by which excess glutamate in the synaptic cleft overstimulates and ultimately kills neurons. This overstimulation is due to lack of transporters to clear glutamate, accumulating and increasing activation of glutamate receptors on neurons. In **epilepsy**, is reduced by changes in expression and function of glutamate receptors, transporters, and enzymes involved in the regulation of glutamate levels. These changes can lead to an imbalance in the levels of glutamate in the synaptic cleft, causing seizures and other symptoms of epilepsy.

In **depression** release and reuptake changes alters signaling and disrupt the activity of brain regions in mood regulation, such as the *prefrontal cortex* and the *amygdala*.

Whether this depends on neurons or glial cells is an important issue. In fact, Glutamatergic astrocytes are a type of glial cell in the central nervous system (CNS) that play an important role in regulating neurotransmission. One of the astrocytes functions, is regulating the concentration of glutamate in the extracellular space and the reuptake of this neurotransmitter.

> Glutamate is the most important neurotransmitter for neuronal excitation in the CNS.

Its release at neuronal synapses is crucial for the transmission of excitatory signals. Glutamatergic astrocytes are equipped with glutamate transporters on their cell membrane, which allow them to remove glutamate from the synaptic space after its release by neurons. This is crucial to prevent **excitotoxicity**, which is a state of neuronal overexcitation caused by excessive levels of glutamate in the brain.

In addition to clearing glutamate from the synaptic space, glutamatergic astrocytes can also convert glutamate into glutamine through an enzyme called glutamine synthetase. Glutamine can be released by astrocytes and taken up by neurons to be converted back into glutamate, allowing for a <mark>recycling cycle of glutamate</mark> that is essential for normal synaptic function.

Maintaining appropriate levels of glutamate in the synaptic space is essential for the health of the central nervous system.

For a life-rich on Glutamate we should consider:

1. Exercise regularly: Exercise has been shown to increase levels of glutamate in the brain, which can improve overall brain function and promote healthy brain plasticity.
2. Eat a balanced diet: Consuming a diet that is rich in nutrients and low in processed foods can support overall brain health and help to maintain healthy levels of glutamate. Foods that are rich in glutamate include salmon, nuts, and eggs.
3. Practice mindfulness and meditation: Regular meditation has been shown to increase glutamate levels in the brain and may also help to improve mood and reduce stress.
4. Get adequate sleep: Sleep is essential for brain function, and a lack of sleep can lead to decreased levels of glutamate in the brain. Aim to get 7-9 hours of sleep each night and practice good sleep hygiene.
5. Stimulate your brain: Engage in activities that challenge your brain and promote learning, such as reading, playing musical instruments, or solving puzzles. These

activities can help to increase the availability of glutamate in the brain and improve overall brain function.

In the whole book you will see that mindfulness meditation and sleep share the effect of increasing any neurotransmitter. Similarly SINGING, improves almost all neurotransmitters: dopamine, endorphins, and oxytocin. But that there are some actions specific for an individual neurotransmitter, in this case they will be presented in de book underlined.

The L-glutamate is an amino-acid neurotransmitter that is produced and used within the brain, and it is not the same as the glutamate in food (monosodium glutamate). Although there is some evidence suggesting that high levels of glutamate in the diet can alter the balance of neurotransmitters in the brain and affect brain function. That is the case of shark fin soup containing high levels of monosodium glutamate (MSG), a sodium salt of glutamic acid, which is one of the 20 amino acids that make up proteins in the body. MSG is a flavor enhancer commonly used in many Asian cuisines. Some people may experience physical symptoms after consuming it, such as headache, flushing, sweating, heart palpitations, and chest pain. These symptoms are commonly referred to as "Chinese restaurant syndrome."
Glutamate is found in many foods: meat, fish, and dairy products. When consumed, it is usually broken down and used as a source of energy or incorporated into other proteins in the body.
There are several types of glutamate receptors, including **ionotropic** glutamate receptors (iGluRs) and **metabotropic** glutamate receptors (mGluRs). iGluRs are ligand-gated ion channels, meaning they allow the flow of ions across the neuronal membrane when glutamate binds to them. Metabotropic glutamate receptors (mGluRs) are G-protein coupled receptors that modulate neuronal activity through intracellular signaling pathways.
The most important ionotropic one is the NMDA or N-methyl-D-aspartate receptors (NMDARs) important for synaptic plasticity and involved in learning and memory processes. They are unique in that they require the simultaneous binding of glutamate and a co-agonist, such as glycine or D-serine, as well as the relief of magnesium blockage, to allow the influx of calcium ions. This calcium influx triggers a cascade of intracellular processes that contribute to long-term potentiation (LTP) and long-term depression (LTD), which are mechanisms underlying synaptic plasticity.
Ionotropic glutamate receptors are involved in quantum spin phenomena within the brain, in other words with quantum mechanical phenomena, specifically the isotope of the gas xenon, xenon-129, which has nuclear spin ½, blocks NMDA receptors producing an anesthetic effect. Nuclear spinless xenon (ie, xenon-128, xenon-130, xenon-132, etc.) does not have the same anesthetic properties.

GABA (gamma-aminobutyric acid) is a neurotransmitter in the central nervous system that functions as an INHIBITORY neurotransmitter. It plays a crucial role in regulating neuronal excitability throughout the brain.

GABA is primarily produced in the brain, specifically in the neurons. It is synthesized **from glutamate**, another neurotransmitter, through a process called decarboxylation. The enzyme glutamate decarboxylase (GAD) facilitates this conversion, leading to the production of GABA. Once synthesized, GABA is released into the synapses between neurons, where it binds to GABA receptors and helps inhibit or reduce the activity of surrounding neurons.

The production and release of GABA help regulate and balance the overall excitatory activity in the brain, contributing to the maintenance of normal brain function and the control of various processes such as anxiety, stress response, and motor control.

DOPAMINERGIC LIFE

Dopamine is produced in various regions of the brain by the dopaminergic neurons, as the ones in the *substantia nigra* and the *hypothalamus* acting as neurotransmitter. When release in the synapsis activate post synaptic neurons binding only 5 types of receptors; the D1 and D2 are the ones related with its reward effects. Dopamine is also produced in the gut by enteric neurons and is involved in regulating gut motility, sensation, and secretions.

Here are the five dopamine receptors and some of their functions:

- D1 receptor: in various regions of the brain (striatum, prefrontal cortex-PFC, and hippocampus). Increase cAMP (cyclic adenosine monophosphate) signaling, increasing excitation and improving working memory, attention, and motivation.
- D2 receptor: the most abundant dopamine receptor in the brain. It is found in many regions (striatum, limbic system, and PFC). Decrease cAMP, decrease excitation and reward-seeking and increase motivation for goal-directed behavior. It is also the receptor on gut Dopamine, located in smooth muscle cells and inhibiting gut motility, modulating gut sensation and secretion. In sensory nerve fibers it inhibit neurotransmitters involved in pain and inflammation, reducing nausea, vomiting, and abdominal pain.
- D3 receptor: found in the mesolimbic and mesocortical areas of the brain. It is involved in motivation and reward processing. Has been implicated in addiction, schizophrenia and depression.
- D4 receptor: mainly found in the PFC, which is involved in decision-making and executive function. It has been linked to attention and impulse control, as well as various neuropsychiatric disorders, including ADHD and bipolar disorder.
- D5 receptor: found in limbic system and cortex. Some studies suggest that it may participate in learning and memory, as well as motivation and reward-seeking behavior.

Dopamine in the brain has important functions, including mood, movement control, motivation, and reward-driven behavior. When it increases under hypnosis also play a role reducing anxiety and stress.

We live searching the way to increase our dopamine because as we will see in the next point it is **the chemical of PURSUIT** and pursuit means actively doing nothing. It increases thinking or fighting for the FUTURE success or reward. And REWARD goes with Win, with to Take something. To be hooked in this scheme forced us to live in the future and not in the present as it should be, because as we will see the reward is short and with several drawbacks.

==Present is the only moment in where we are BEINGS.==

Take into consideration high-dopamine level of the *falling-in-love* period. When we experience feelings of love, the brain releases high levels of Dopamine, leading to feelings of euphoria, increased energy, and a heightened focus on the loved one. This creates a positive feedback loop, as the pleasurable feelings associated with dopamine release reinforce the behavior that led to its release in the first place, further strengthening feelings of love. However, it is worth noting that the intense feelings associated with the *falling-in-love* period are not necessarily indicative of a long-lasting, healthy relationship, and that the dopamine levels may decrease over time as the relationship progresses. As we will see _falling-in-love is a Dopamine addition_ and an abrupt stop produce an abstinence syndrome. On the other hand, people deep bonding with a long-lasting love is associated with an Oxytocin predominant life.

Dopamine is the neurotransmitter of the PLEASURE that carry the phenomenon of REWARD.

When the reward is obtained, the sense of pleasure is giving by the **EOPs** (Endogenous opioid peptides), specifically beta-endorphin, enkephalin and dynorphin. This are the opioids that create an addition.

This means that when you feel pleasure you want more.

Neurotransmitters are so important that neurons are specialized in recapture those molecules that have not been used during a dopamine shot.

A deficiency or low levels of dopamine can result in several diseases, including:

- Parkinson's disease: This is a degenerative disorder of the nervous system that is characterized by tremors, rigidity, and difficulty with movement.
- Attention Deficit Hyperactivity Disorder (ADHD): ADHD is a neurodevelopmental disorder characterized by inattention, hyperactivity, and impulsivity and directly related with re-capture failure of Dopamine.
- Depression: Depression is a mental health disorder characterized by feelings of sadness, hopelessness, and a lack of motivation.
- Schizophrenia: This is a severe mental health disorder that affects how a person thinks, feels, and behaves.
- Addiction: Dopamine is involved in the reward pathways of the brain, and a deficiency in dopamine can contribute to addiction...

At the beginning of this chapter, we mention that DOPAMINE plus ENDORPHINES produce addiction, and as you see in the above paragraph Addiction is one of the main drawbacks of dopamine system because it has an essential role in the reward pathways. And the same can be say of other dopamine agonists as the **Cocaine** or opioid agonists as the **Heroin**.

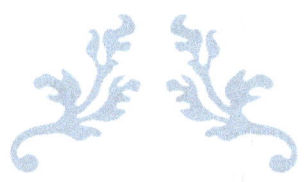

We have several reward pathways in the brain, including the mesolimbic dopamine pathway, the hypothalamic-pituitary-adrenal (HPA) axis, and the endocannabinoid system. They work together to regulate the brain's response to pleasure and emotions, motivation, and reward-seeking behavior.

Be aware that CHRONIC EXCESSIVE REWARD depletes those systems and leads to ADDITION and DEPRESSION. Under the deficit of healthy internal stimulants people often substituted them by external products (drugs, alcohol...) or aberrant philias.

The **mesolimbic dopamine pathway** is integrated by a group of interconnected brain structures such as the *ventral tegmental area (VTA)*, the *nucleus accumbens (NAc)*, and the *prefrontal* cortex (PFC). These structures work together to regulate feelings of pleasure and reward. The release of dopamine activating the NAc is the key aspect of the brain's reward system, as it helps to reinforce behavior that is linked to the experience of pleasure (learning path) through **the EOPs (endogenous opioid peptides)** that are like heroin or morphine. The sensations of pleasure that EOPs generate at reward consummation are **internal experiences**.
There are therefore two nuclei and two functions: VTA is where Dopamine neurons are, it is the motivation area, where impulses of the primitive brain not under control stimulate the dendrite receptors in the NA; the NA is where EOPs neurons are, thanks to which we feel internally pleasure depending of the number of receptors genetically determined being accustomed and creating addition.

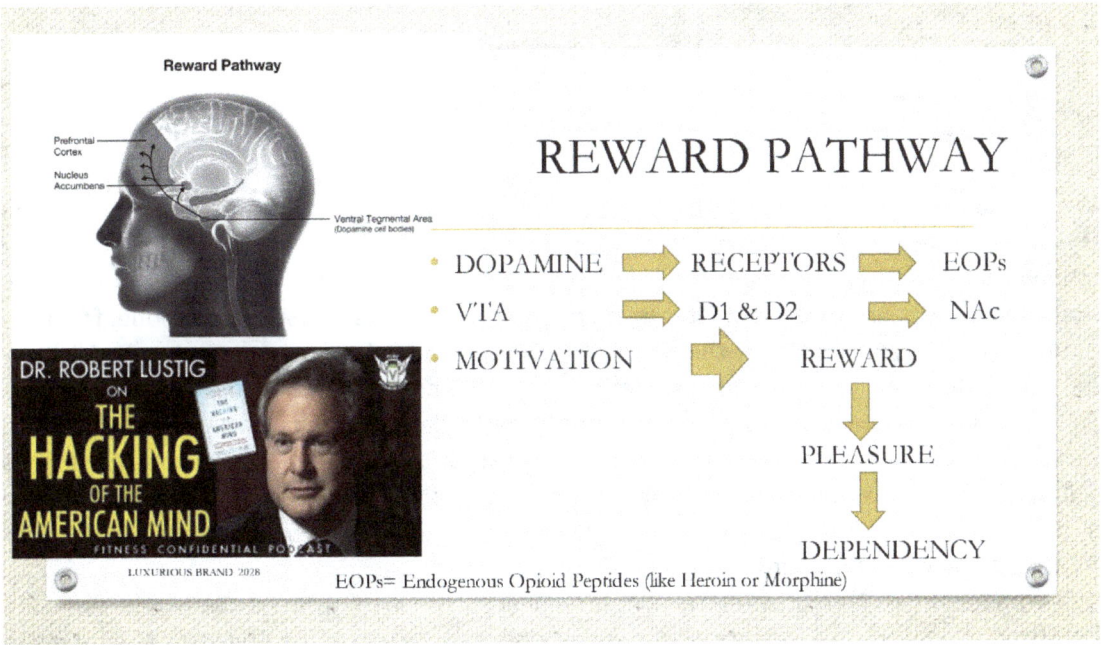

The **endocannabinoid system (ECS)** is a biological system of neurotransmitters and receptors, present throughout the body (brain, liver, pancreas, and reproductive organs, among others) They are produced in various cells, including neurons, immune cells, adipocytes (fat cells), and glial cells of the type of astrocytes and microglia, the latter the immune system of the brain. The ECS plays a role in regulating various physiological and cognitive processes. Among the physiological processes beyond the nervous system, metabolism, inflammation, and immune function. Among the cognitive processes pain, appetite, mood, and memory. The most well-known endocannabinoids are anandamide and 2-arachidonoylglycerol (2-AG).

By contrast Endorphins, as explained in the specific section, are located in the brain being neurotransmitters that act as pain inhibitors and mood elevators. They bind to specific receptors in the brain and produce a feeling of euphoria and pain relief. They are produced in response to stress, exercise, and other stimuli and are involved in regulating pain, stress, and other physiological processes.

Both the ECS and endorphins have pain-relieving properties, but they are separate and distinct systems.

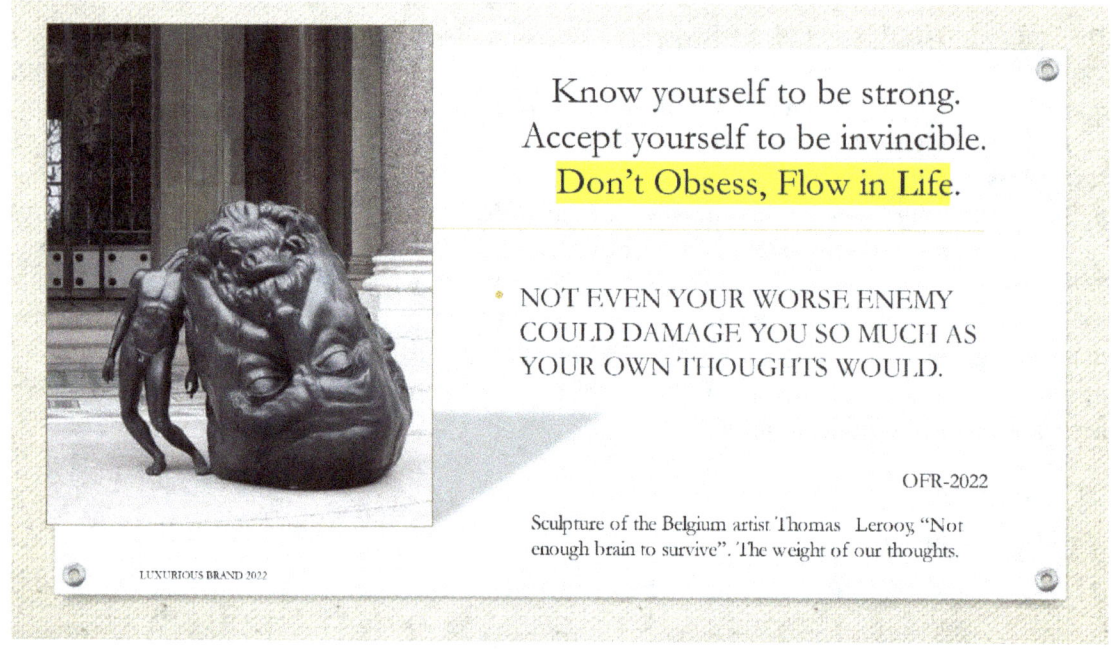

Know yourself to be strong.
Accept yourself to be invincible.
Don't Obsess, Flow in Life.

· NOT EVEN YOUR WORSE ENEMY COULD DAMAGE YOU SO MUCH AS YOUR OWN THOUGHTS WOULD.

OFR-2022

Sculpture of the Belgium artist Thomas Lerooy, "Not enough brain to survive". The weight of our thoughts.

LUXURIOUS BRAND 2022

We should care about the third reward system, the so called **hypothalamic-pituitary-adrenal (HPA) axis**, because it releases stress hormones in response to stressors. The HPA axis influences *reward-seeking behaviors*, and regulates mood, energy levels, and motivation. Activated in response to stressors it triggers the release of cortisol, a stress hormone, from the adrenal gland. Cortisol acts on the brain to increase motivation and energy levels, allowing individuals to respond to the stressor effectively. When cortisol is released in response to stress, it interacts with receptors in the brain, particularly in areas involved in mood and motivation. Cortisol can increase alertness, arousal, and focus, which can contribute to a temporary boost in energy and motivation. However, prolonged activation of the HPA reward system can lead to CHRONIC STRESS and negative health effects, such as decreased mood and motivation, and produced anxiety and depression.

The component of chronic stress is a determining factor in "**Chronopathy**" when someone consistently engages in excessive work (workalcoholism), stress, and a drive to optimize every minute. It is possible that it can result in chronic activation of the stress response, including the HPA axis. When the HPA axis is constantly stimulated, it can disrupt the body's natural balance and potentially lead to various health problems. These may include fatigue, sleep disturbances, weakened immune function, increased risk of anxiety and depression, to reach the "**burnout syndrome**". It is important to find a balance between productivity and self-care. Allowing time for rest, relaxation, and rejuvenation is crucial for overall well-being. Managing stress levels, setting boundaries, and prioritizing self-care activities can help prevent the chronic activation of the HPA axis and reduce the risk of negative health effects associated with excessive stress and productivity.

Other hormones are not strange to the motivation system, this is the case of ESTROGENS. Increase estrogens means increase dopamine. That is one of the reasons of the change of humor in women. During the first part of the cycle estrogen raised and arrive to the peak on ovulation (dopamine do the same) after that, estrogen starts to drop (as dopamine) and mood become worse, more aggressive and without motivation. I always thought that since this did not happen in men, maybe is a natural trick to maintain motivation in a couple avoiding getting bored.

First the MOTIVATION and then the consummation with the PLEASURE.

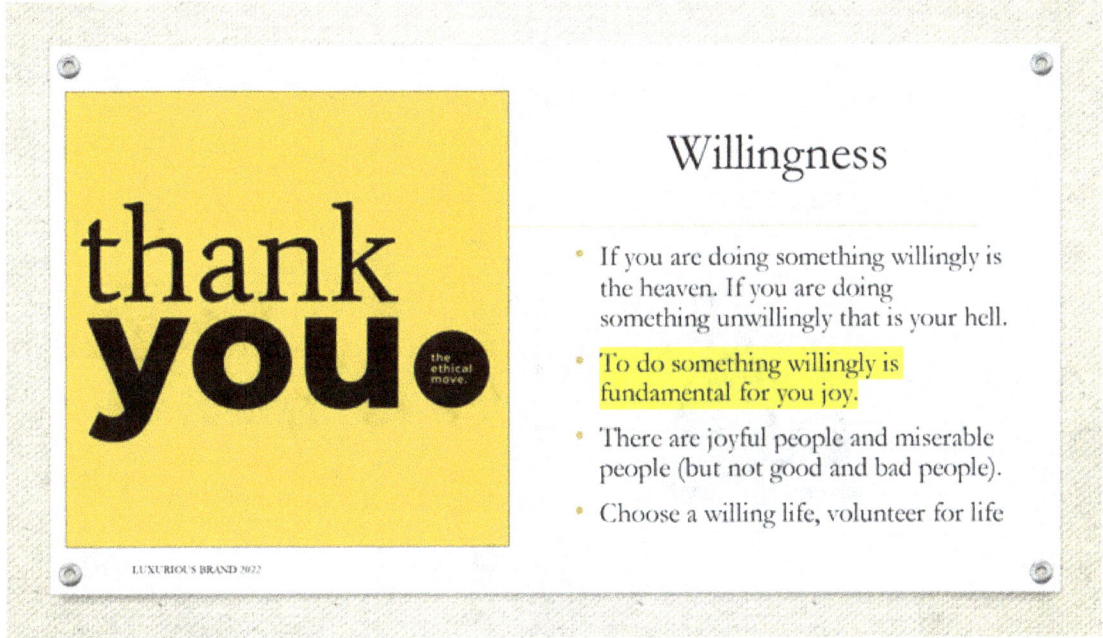

The good people (see EGO chapter) are an integration of virtues that help them **cultivate a valuable life**, not only for themselves, but for the others. Being good does not only imply stopping doing evil or avoiding falling into it, being good is a **willingness to act actively in life**, (MOTIVATION) always seeking to favor its development at all levels.

After these definitions you probably will ask yourself and **where is the AMBITION**?
Ambition is never a problem, ambition is a motor, is the motivation to bring you to the goal, but this goal must be outside oneself not linked to your EGO, not linked to your internal feeling of pleasure. The customers, the family, the friends, the society, the environment, the quality of life... those are goals that must guide you and that will make you to feel you happy thanks to Serotonin.

If you do not use your passion to create self-fulfillment, the ambition will destroy you.

You already know the reason; you will get trapped in the reward system and become dependent.
Change urgently your focus and your goal. Assure that YOUR WIN is to benefit others and that is not linked with EOPs, meaning with internal opioids, with internal pleasure, with your Ego; on the contrary, it is linked with external achievements, people's help, love to others, in summary that what you gain is an oxytocin and serotonin shot.

Serotonin can reset the dopamine system. This reset occurs through a process called DESENSITIZATION, where repeated exposure to a neurotransmitter leads to a decrease in its effectiveness. When the activity of dopamine-releasing neurons is increased, the release of serotonin from other neurons is also increased. This increase in serotonin causes a decrease in the sensitivity of dopamine receptors, leading to a reset of the dopamine system, for your good, moving you away from the dependency.

Never forget that in the simplicity of life is where happiness and peacefulness are found.

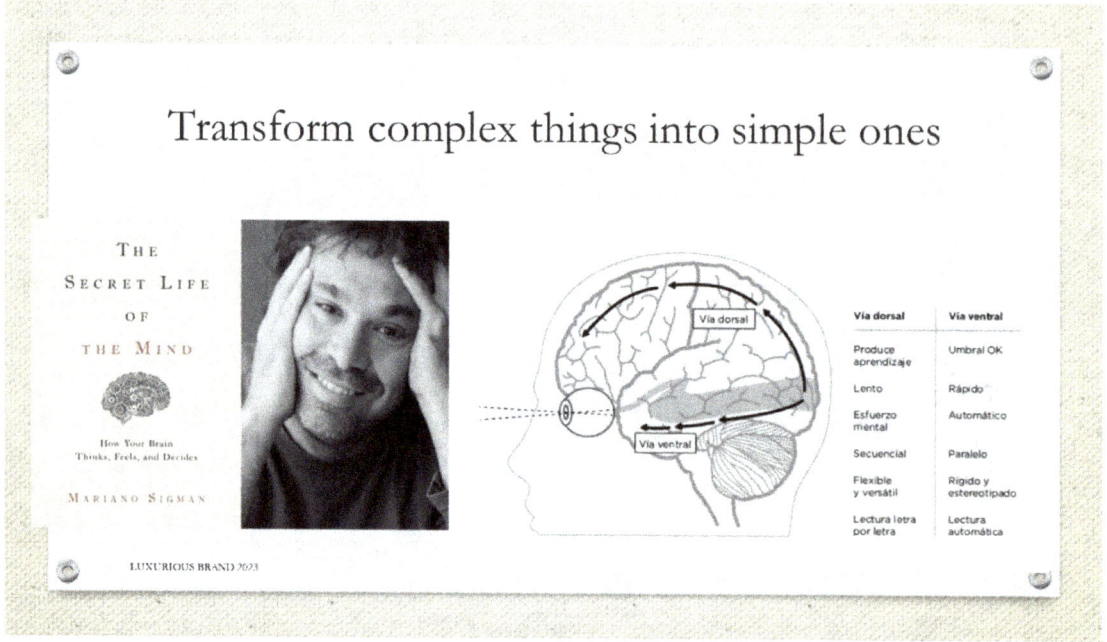

Simplicity is the sacred grail of intelligent people. Only very intelligent people can transform complex tasks into simple ones. And our brain learns and becomes efficient in the same way, changing the path from the dorsal to the ventral route. Simplifying, automating in the ventral path those that we have repeat with effort, motivation, and patience through the dorsal path. We learn increasing our consciousness until the level it become simple, unconscious (we enter into the self-hypnotic loop explained in chapter one), part of ourselves carrying out a parallel computing neuronal path prepared to be activated next time.

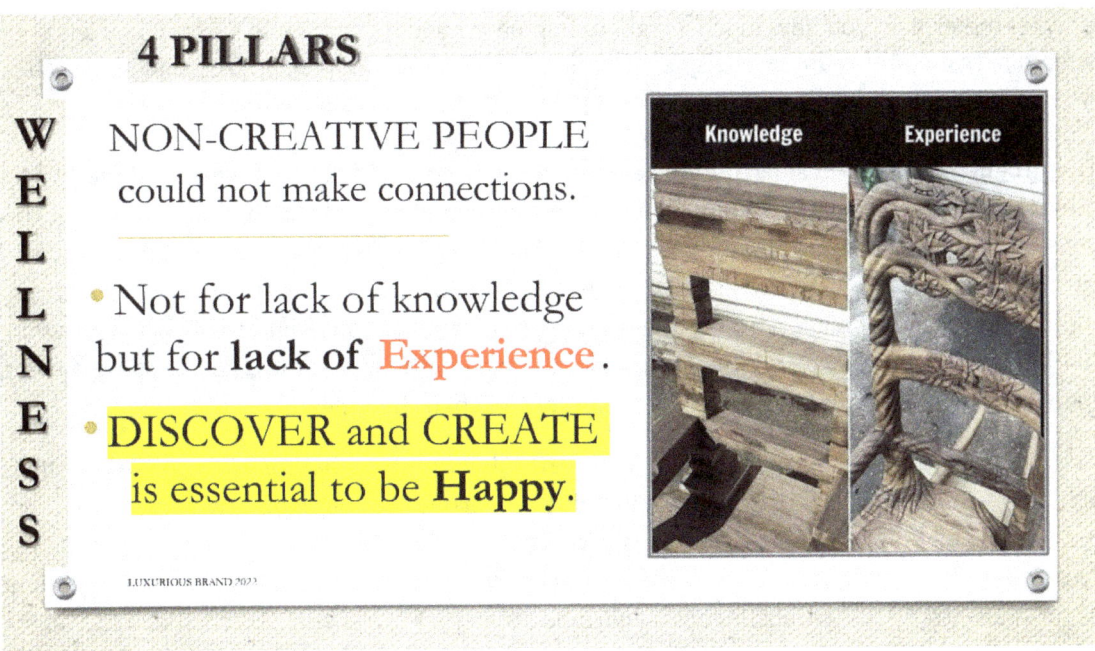

4 PILLARS

W E L L N E S S

NON-CREATIVE PEOPLE could not make connections.

• Not for lack of knowledge but for **lack of Experience**.

• DISCOVER and CREATE is essential to be **Happy**.

Knowledge / Experience

LUXURIOUS BRAND 2023

Discover and create is essential to be happy. And this cannot be achieved without effort, motivation, and patience.

To be motivated we need and produce DOPAMINE.

That is the reason why people lacking Dopamine as in Attention Deficit (ADHD), only get focus, attentive and learn when they find something that motivate them. In other word a generalized principle for learning activity.

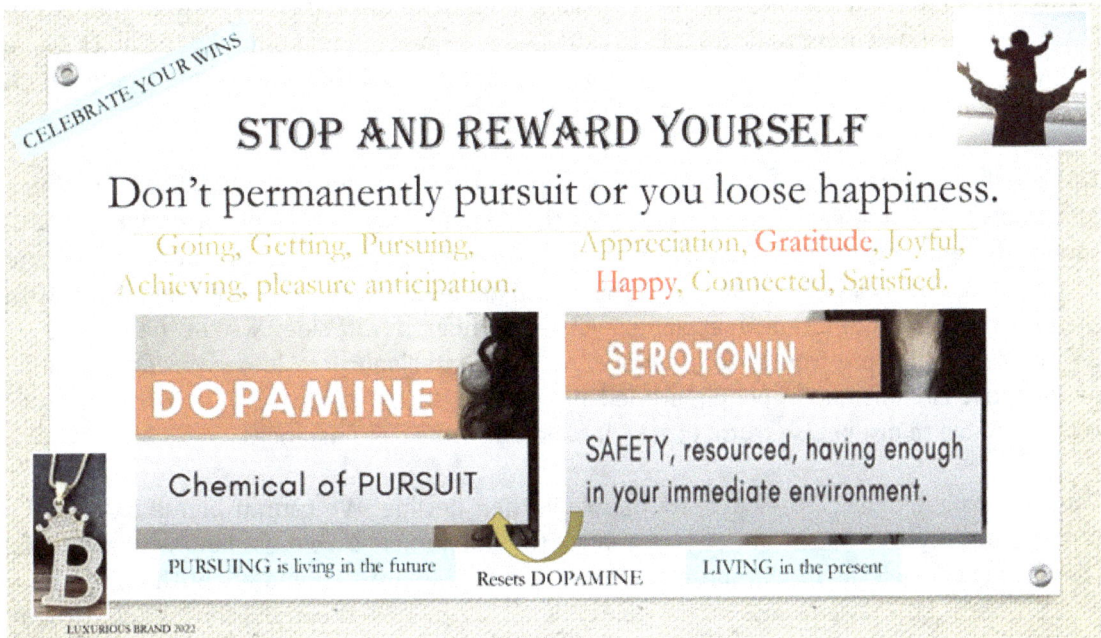

CELEBRATE YOUR WINS

STOP AND REWARD YOURSELF

Don't permanently pursuit or you loose happiness.

Going, Getting, Pursuing, Achieving, pleasure anticipation.

Appreciation, Gratitude, Joyful, Happy, Connected, Satisfied.

DOPAMINE — Chemical of PURSUIT

SEROTONIN — SAFETY, resourced, having enough in your immediate environment.

PURSUING is living in the future — Resets DOPAMINE — LIVING in the present

LUXURIOUS BRAND 2022

DOPAMINE PLAY

Now let me explain you how much we get manipulated when people and society play with our dopaminergic system, up to the level that finally people cannot recognize what is fake and what is truth. When you hear enough lies you are not able to recognize the truth at all.

The **drogue of "likes"** in smartphone screens. Social media and screens **were designed to be addictive**, to produce a feeling of wellness in our mind and were developed just to exploit this vulnerability of humans to create addiction. Nothing make us to feel better that to understand that we are loved, appreciated, that the rest of people care by our things. This is a strong motivation, like an addiction from the hormone point of view. Consumption of cocaine, heroin, marihuana, alcohol, have sex, view pornography, play with videogames, go shopping, have a meal with friends…, all produce pleasure, ones better than the others.

And pleasure is regulated in our brain by several hormones, but particularly **DOPAMINE**. Dopamine starts to raise just planning the idea to perpetrate the action, whatever it is, that produce us pleasure. When the action is accomplished **the abstinence syndrome** raised. The fact is that for every "like" you received in social media there is a shot of Dopamine in your brain and afterwards an abstinence syndrome, that make you feel depressed, lost, angry, empty… if there is no interior life that maintain you in the present, building life, just BEING.

To understand how true this is, here is a storytelling. Have you ever thought why the biggest heads in IT and social media DO NOT ALLOW their children to access the screens (Steve Jobs, Bill Gates, …) Most of them sign contracts with their Nannies in which there is a clause that do not allow them to have mobiles or screens when working with their children. They are as drogue traffickers which principles is: "NEVER CONSUME; be the others the ones to consume to make me reach".

Problem raises **particularly in children**, who sometimes in their lives (8-12 years) they will have an IDENTITY CRISIS (hormone, psychical, social change) and a frustration. At that moment to know how to **handle bore and stress** is essential, and children should not take the quick scape of social media. That is the reason why it is advised not to allow to use social media before 12, or in general before or during adolescence crisis.

The problem is huge, our Pre-frontal zone carry out the attention, concentration, problem resolution and impulse control. If you know that babies only fixed their attention to **light, sound and movement** you would immediately understand how attractive social medial and audio-visual tools will be for babies and children in general. If you know that brain works with the principle: "use it or lose it" (I explained you, remember, during sleep we cut the sprouts we do not need), the pre-frontal zone where the main intelligence resides is losing potential; under those circumstances, people are led to fakes, to show leadership at any cost in social media, unable to distinguish truth, totally dominated by the circumstances.

They are drogue-addicts, they are sick people in their decline. **We cannot blame individually but as a society**. We must find tools to control the phenomena, we must help with solutions: (1) those that are legal and business model compatible, so firms should adopt them (2) those that are legal but not business model compatible, so firms need compulsion to adopt them, and (3) those that require changes to bad law.

Dependencies to Dopamine are everywhere, one example is fun TATTO making. Getting a tattoo can activate a variety of neurotransmitters and neuropeptides, such as endorphins, adrenaline, and dopamine. Endorphins, released in response to pain and stress, can create feelings of pleasure and euphoria. Adrenaline can create a feeling of excitement and energy in the body. Dopamine is released just planning the meaningful and enjoyable experience that tattoo represent for some people, when finished (the win) dopamine give a sense of pleasure that together with endorphin produce dependency.

More worrisome is their relationship with <u>FANATICISM and extremism</u>. In the context of belief and fanaticism, dopamine reinforces and strengthen our convictions and sense of identity. When we encounter information or experiences that confirm our beliefs, our brain releases dopamine, which gives us a sense of pleasure and reward. This can create a positive feedback loop where we seek out more information that confirms our beliefs and avoid information that contradicts them. Over time, this can lead to a strong emotional attachment to our beliefs and a sense of identity tied to them. When our beliefs are challenged or threatened, our brain may respond with stress and anxiety, which can lead to defensive or even aggressive responses. This can be especially true for beliefs that are tied to our sense of identity or social group, such as religious or political beliefs.

And in political beliefs (but also in religion) we are seeking the pleasure produce by a Dopamine shot. In extreme cases, this pattern of reinforcement and identity can lead to fanaticism, where individuals become highly devoted and even obsessed with their beliefs. They may be willing to engage in extreme or even violent behaviors to defend their beliefs, as their brain's reward system reinforces this behavior as highly pleasurable and rewarding.

> In politics everything we do have this premise, have to be pleasurable and rewarding.

It is important to note that dopamine is just one factor that can contribute to fanaticism, and that there are many complex psychological, social, and cultural factors that can influence belief and identity. You can find more in CULTURAL CONDITIONING chapter and in the EGO chapter. Nevertheless, these tendencies try to lower down with age for reasons such as:

1. Increased life experience: As people age, they tend to have more life experiences and exposure to different perspectives and ideas. This can broaden their understanding of the world and make them more tolerant and accepting of diversity.
2. Greater cognitive flexibility: As people age, their brains become less rigid and more adaptable to new information and perspectives.
3. Changes in motivation: As people age, their priorities and values may shift, and they may become less focused on defending their beliefs or seeking validation from others.
4. Reduced social pressure: As people age, they may become less concerned with social status or peer pressure, which can make it easier for them to challenge conventional wisdom and think independently.
5. Improved emotional regulation: As people age, they tend to develop better emotional regulation skills, which can help them avoid becoming overly attached to their beliefs or reacting defensively to challenging ideas or perspectives.

As we mentioned, a DOPAMINE life brings you to live in the FUTURE, searching-pursuing pleasure and reaching an abstinence syndrome when the Dopamine shot (pleasure episodes) finishes because when you get the final reward your opioid system is released. Therefore, is not always good to choose to have a dopaminergic life with things such as:

1. Pursuit goals and achieve them: Setting and achieving goals can give you a sense of accomplishment and release dopamine, making you feel more motivated and satisfied. Set achievable goals and plans to achieve them, focusing on progress, not perfection. But keep in mind that your goals should not be based on your EGO.
2. Engage in physical activity: Physical activity has been shown to increase dopamine levels in the brain, making it a great way to enhance motivation and improve mood.

Try to incorporate exercise into your daily routine, such as going for a walk, lifting weights, or participating in team sports.

3. Seek new experiences: Trying new things can be a great way to increase dopamine levels and boost motivation. Try new foods, travel to new places, or take up new hobbies to keep life interesting and engaging.

4. Seek people that bring you joy: Seek out relationships with people who bring positivity and joy into your life. The extreme is to *fall-in-love*.

5. Get enough sleep: Sleep is important for regulating mood and overall well-being, and poor sleep can decrease dopamine levels. Try to get 7-9 hours of sleep each night and establish a consistent sleep schedule.

6. Practice gratitude: Focusing on what you are grateful for, this increase dopamine and improve mood. Take a few minutes each day to find what you are thankful for and to express gratitude. GRATITUDE as we already mention is infective.

7. Engage in pleasurable activities: Engaging in activities that you find enjoyable, such as hobbies, spending time with friends, or listening to music, can release dopamine and boost motivation.

It is very significant that people with deficit of Dopamine are very competitive, as it happens in the Attention Deficit ADHD. The engagement for a future reward in competition is a wide fountain of dopamine for them, being highly frustrated if they do not win.

The real life (to live in the PRESENT) is the only one that allow us to produce SEROTONIN and OXYTOCIN. Serotonin with the feeling of happiness and accomplishment. Oxytocin with love, kisses, time spend, nature and sports sharing as we will see latter on.

If you are looking for a DOPAMINERGIC LIFE, stay on the motivation and shift to the SEROTONIN LIFE to achieved self-fulfillment and not internal pleasure for a personal reward.

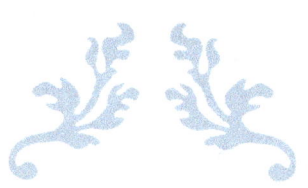

Serotonin is a neurotransmitter involved in the regulation of mood, appetite, and sleep. It is primarily produced in the *Dorsal Raphe Nucleus (DRN)* of the brainstem going through multiple parts of the brain creating numerous experiences and judgements. The complexity of Serotonin receptors is high, with at least 14 different types acting in the brain, expression of the numerous Serotonin responses most of them unknown, that we will study latter on. Hypnosis also increases serotonin levels in the brain and help to induce a state of deep relaxation reducing pain perception.

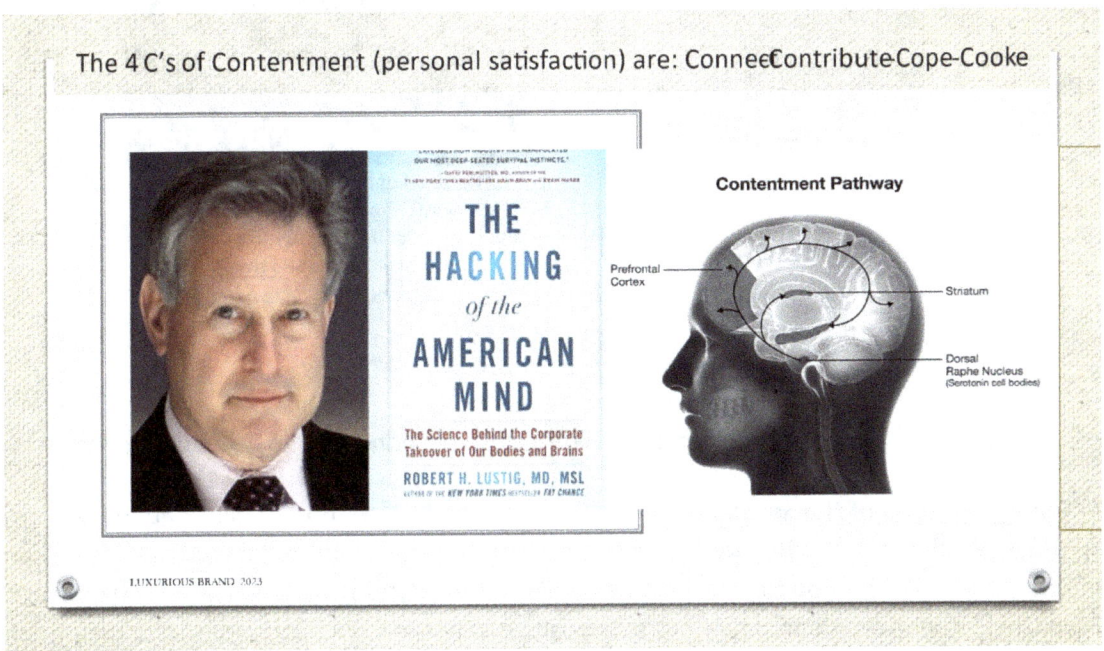

The 4 C's of Contentment (personal satisfaction) are: Connec-Contribute-Cope-Cooke

Serotonin is known as the **hormone of HAPPINESS**. It generates feelings of well-being, relaxation, satisfaction, bonding, increases concentration and self-esteem. Serotonin is a neurotransmitter that plays a key role in regulating mood (our MOOD STABILIZER), cognition, perception, and other aspects of brain function. It is Serotonin-1a receptor the one in charge of subjective well-being, serenity, eudemonia and containment. As we studied, Serotonin is considered responsible for the astral flights induced by the DMT that bring a sense of connection to a spiritual realm and it is Serotonin-2a receptor the one in charge of that mystical experiences. Whatever is felt with Serotonin it occurs in the PRESENT.

It increases with gratitude, satisfaction, joyfulness, appreciation, connectivity, go to nature...

Is the neurotransmitter of HAPPINESS that incorporate CONTENTMENT and FULFILLMENT.

This means that when you are happy you are self-satisfied and do not want anything else. And this is unrelated to the circumstances.

Maybe this definition could allow you to understand how in the extreme fulfillment obtained by overstimulation of the Serotonin system, our internal-self does reach the understanding of God, goes to our superior spiritual realm, our Infinite Consciousness, because the individual is in a total plenitude. From the pragmatic point of view, it represents that when Serotonin receptor-1a is full and the neurotransmitter goes to Serotonin receptor-2a.

It also clarifies that Serotonin is the MAIN MOOD provider and therefore mood disorders are linked to this neurotransmitter.

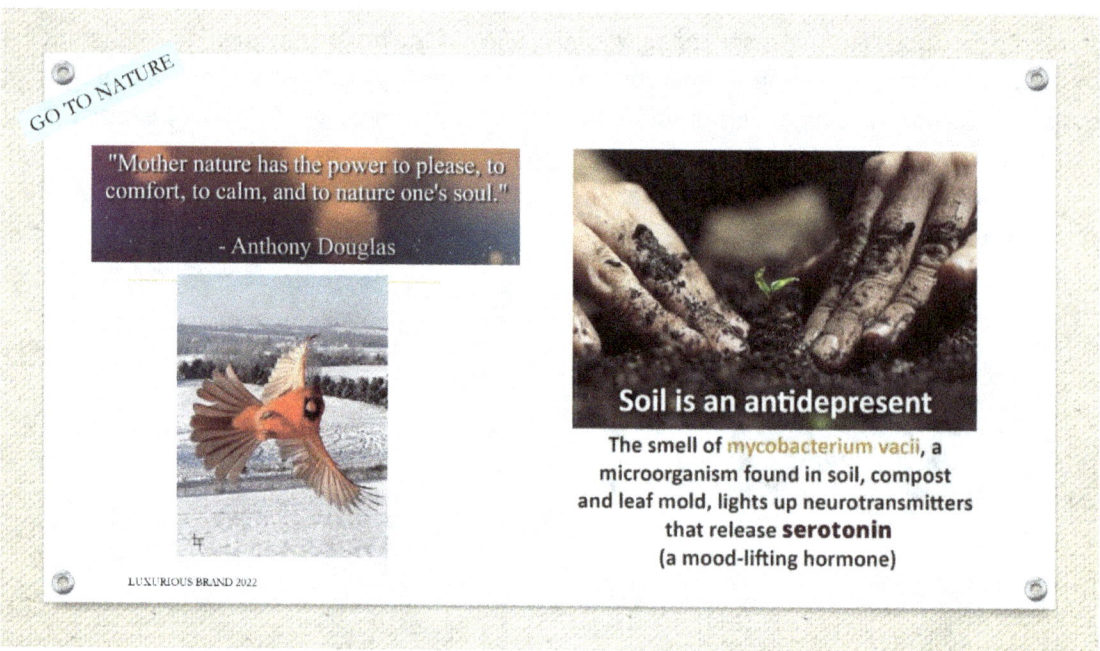

"Mother nature has the power to please, to comfort, to calm, and to nature one's soul."
- Anthony Douglas

GO TO NATURE

LUXURIOUS BRAND 2022

Soil is an antidepresent

The smell of mycobacterium vacii, a microorganism found in soil, compost and leaf mold, lights up neurotransmitters that release **serotonin** (a mood-lifting hormone)

==When we go to the nature, we also feel this sense of connection to a spiritual realm.==

In **Overstimulation** of the Serotonin system, our sensorial perceptions, hallucinations, visions, spiritual realities, astral trips produce high level of happiness and fulfillment; we are in an internal feeling that nothing else is needed, and everything is beauty and happiness. Nevertheless, not everyone pours out in a positive way their own consciousness, their Soul; some people project negative and destructive entities as we will see in the Serotonin syndrome section below.

We stated previously that "we are what our neurotransmitters allow us to be", and they can be manipulated sometimes for good, sometimes for bad.

➤ For Good: It is clearly demonstrated that RELIGION (whatever) impacts your Serotonin level and creates containment. Now is time to think whether it is your self-consciousness who brings you to God, because He is within you, and you are part of something bigger than yourself.

Most religions also promote social connection and social good to get happiness and self-satisfaction for what you do for others. This may let you think that all religions are extensible comparable, they are created by similar or dissimilar human minds, because whatever is God, whatever is the World's intelligence, It is in you. The energy of your several consciousness will be transformed -when the substrate (neurons) disappears- into the Infinity Consciousness in another not yet known energy (electromagnetic, autopoietic, coded…) capable or not to be detected, to evolve, to transform, to maintain individual self-consciousness or to reincarnate. People with high serotonin, related or not with religious feelings, are not afraid to die. And in some spiritual eastern religions when they arrive to the maximum happiness and fulfillment by meditation they seek to die and really die by mean of fasting.

Self-transcendence and spiritual acceptance involve Serotonin in DRN (serotonin neurons), following hippocampus (memory) and cortex (processing thoughts) and its religiosity is genetic determined by the type of 1a-receptors. Furthermore, expert consider that is Dopamine the trigger that transform believers into fanatics and extremists' religious people as we explainrd in the Dopamine section.

> For bad: Some people with practices that involve altered states of consciousness, such as meditation, lucid dreaming, or the use of psychedelic substances, obtain bad experiences. People with a history of trauma or mental health issues may be more vulnerable to negative experiences as well as people who are feeling stressed or anxious. Another possible explanation is the nature of the practice or substance being used. For example, some psychedelic substances can induce challenging or difficult experiences, sometimes referred to as "bad trips," which can be emotionally intense and difficult to manage. Similarly, certain types of meditation or spiritual practices may involve confronting and working through difficult emotions or past traumas, which can be challenging and overwhelming.

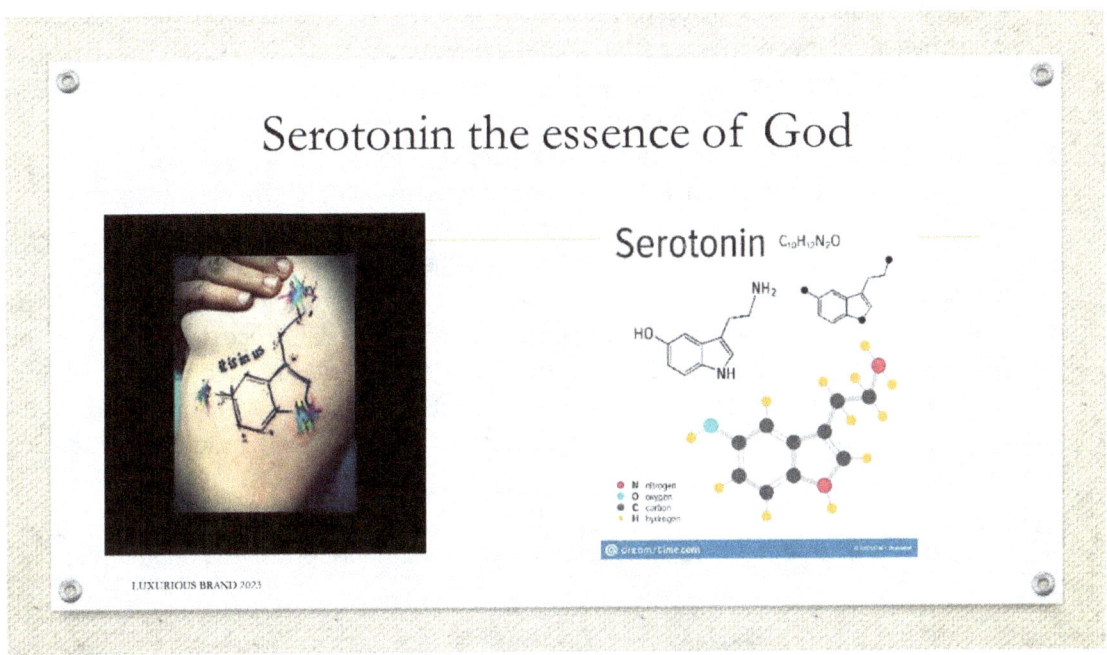

Serotonin structure was confirmed in 1953, and psychotropic substances specifically LSD and Psylocibin have incredible similarities binding specifically serotonin 1a-receptors (containment function) and 2a-receptors (mystical experiences-metaphysical trips). The tryptamine psychedelics (LSD and Psylocibin) stimulate first 2a-receptors and after the mystic experience the 1a-receptor feeling containment. Mescaline on the contrary only binds 2a-receptors while MDMA not only binds 2a-receptors but also dopamine receptors.

Here are some ways you can build a serotonin-rich life:

1. Get sunlight exposure: Sunlight exposure has been shown to increase serotonin levels in the brain. Particularly in the morning when sunlight is most intense. The prolonged lack of sunlight (for example, at the North Pole or during the transition from summer to winter) can cause a transient depressive syndrome, the so-called Seasonal Affective Disorder (SAD) or "Winter Blues". At the other extreme, regions close to the tropics, with their peculiar happy lifestyle, could be due to more sun exposure.

2. Go to the Nature: Be embedded in the magnificence of the Natural world, play with the soil, smell the nature… You have already seen that soil containing *Mycobacterium vacii* produces an odor that stimulates Serotonin.

3. Exercise: Exercise has been shown to boost serotonin levels, as well as improve mood and overall well-being thanks to endorphins and rejuvenates the body as we will see in our next book.

4. Eat a healthy diet: Consuming a diet that is rich in complex carbohydrates, such as fruits, vegetables, and whole grains, increase serotonin levels. Avoid consuming excessive amounts of sugar and processed foods, as these can have a negative impact on mood and well-being deriving is the so-called **Metabolic syndrome** that carries heart disease, stroke, Alzheimer, diabetes and kidney disease. And of which we will extensively cover in the final book of the trilogy.

5. Get enough sleep: Sleep is important for regulating mood and overall well-being, and poor sleep can decrease serotonin levels. Try to get 7-9 hours of sleep each night and establish a consistent sleep schedule.

6. Engage in pleasurable activities: Engaging in activities that you find enjoyable, such as hobbies, spending time with friends, or listening to music, can boost serotonin levels and improve mood.

7. Practice mindfulness: It helps to reduce stress and anxiety and improve overall well-being. Regulate mood and increase serotonin levels.

8. Seek professional help: If you are struggling with symptoms of depression or anxiety. Antidepressant medications can increase serotonin levels and improve mood.

9. Deep breathing exercises have been shown to have a positive effect on neurotransmitter activation in the brain. This is because deep breathing can help regulate the balance of certain neurotransmitters, such as serotonin, which plays a role in regulating mood, appetite, and sleep. When we breathe deeply, we stimulate the *Vagus Nerve*, which is a cranial nerve that runs from the brainstem to the abdomen and is involved in regulating various physiological processes, including the release of neurotransmitters. By activating the Vagus Nerve through deep breathing, we can increase the release of neurotransmitters such as serotonin and GABA (gamma-aminobutyric acid), which are involved in regulating mood and reducing anxiety.

The 4 C's of Contentment (personal satisfaction) are: Connect-Contribute-Cope-Cooke

---

Regarding breathing there is a connection with the neurotransmitter function. Different types of breathing can have different effects on neurotransmitters, which can impact your physical and mental well-being. For example, slow, deep breathing has been shown to activate the parasympathetic nervous system, which can help to reduce stress and anxiety. This type of breathing has been shown to increase levels of GABA, a neurotransmitter that has calming effects on the body and mind.

Breathing through the nose, as opposed to the mouth, has been shown to have an impact on the brain, not only by the close location of the nose roof to the base of the brain (sniffed drugs enter the blood stream in the highly vascularized nose mucosae and go directly to the brain). Nasal breathing has been linked to higher levels of NITRIC OXIDE (NO), a molecule that acts as a neurotransmitter and has many beneficial effects on the body, including reducing inflammation and promoting relaxation.

➤ The NO is involved in a variety of physiological processes in the brain, including learning and memory, pain modulation, and regulation of blood flow. Dysregulation of NO signaling has been implicated in a number of neurological and psychiatric disorders, including Alzheimer's disease, Parkinson's disease, and depression. The overall effect of NO as a neurotransmitter is to enhance or inhibit the release of other neurotransmitters, depending on the specific receptors and signaling pathways involved.

➤ The NO is a gas. Unlike traditional neurotransmitters stored in vesicles and released from presynaptic neurons, the NO is produced on demand in the postsynaptic neuron and diffuses across the synaptic cleft to affect the presynaptic neuron. When an action potential reaches the postsynaptic neuron, it triggers the activation of an enzyme called nitric oxide synthase (NOS), which converts arginine into NO. The NO then diffuses across the synaptic cleft to the presynaptic neuron, where it can bind to and activate guanylate cyclase, an enzyme that produces cyclic guanosine monophosphate (cGMP). cGMP can then trigger a cascade of signaling events within the presynaptic neuron, such as the activation of ion channels or the modulation of neurotransmitter release.

<u>Mouth breathing</u>, by contrary, can have negative effects on neurotransmitter function. For example, it has been linked to a decrease in serotonin, the neurotransmitter regulating mood and promoting feelings of well-being.

<u>Slow breathing</u> can effectively control pain in the following manner. Approximately 10% of amygdala activity can be attributed to the type of breathing, specifically the process of expiration rather than inspiration. Inspiration has a more direct impact on the insula, which is associated with self-identity, the orbitofrontal cortex, linked to relaxation, and the temporal cortex and hippocampus, involved in memory, particularly during nasal inspiration. To activate these areas extensively, breathing should be gentle and slow, with particular emphasis on the duration of expiration to effectively relax the amygdala, which requires twice as much time.

Overall, it appears that the type and rate of breathing can have significant effects on neurotransmitter function, and that different types of breathing can be used to support different aspects of mental and physical health.

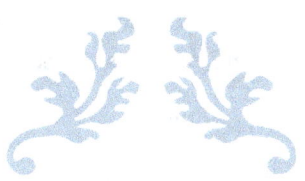

The source of human Serotonin and Dopamine is not only the brain, they are also produced in the gut. The gut is often referred to as the "**SECOND BRAIN**" due to its complex network of neurons, which can produce and release neurotransmitters. Serotonin is synthesized by enterochromaffin cells in the gut and plays a role in regulating gut motility and the sensation of fullness and hunger that control the appetite.

In fact, the majority of serotonin in the body is found in the gastrointestinal tract, and although the blood-brain barrier helps to regulate the transfer of substances, some serotonin can cross the barrier and enter the brain, where it can then affect mood, appetite, and other functions. This contrast with the dopamine that some may be found in the gut, but which main source in the body is the brain, and furthermore in this case it is not clear if abdominal dopamine can cross the barrier to enter the brain.

Serotonin and dopamine contribute to various gastrointestinal disorders, such as irritable bowel syndrome and inflammatory bowel disease. Additionally, changes in levels can affect mood, stress, and other aspects of brain function, highlighting the close relationship between the gut and the brain.

The **gut microbiome** refers to the collection of bacteria and other microorganisms that live in the gut and are important for overall health. They are in charge to produce and release various neurotransmitters, including serotonin, dopamine, and GABA, which play a role in regulating mood and behavior.

Whether the Second Brain is the one that bring us one of two most important senses such an interception and proprioception can be discussed. Interception includes information gaining the brain from our internal body (heart, brain, intestine...). Proprioception is the information that arrive to our brain from our external personal body (posture, gesture, sensations...). Our memory conscious or unconscious come from everywhere in the body and everything outside.

Bear in mind that ALL BODY is a lifelong memory that influences our world perception and create our world. Not only our brain remembers, is the whole body that remembers.

- Our SKIN remembers (touches, people, lovers, sensations, wind, speed...

- Our GUT remembers (fear, love, stress, food, disgust, sickness...

- Our MOUTH remembers (savors, caress, thirsty, food, disgust, kisses...

- Our LEGS remember (runs, cycle, efforts, weakness, mountains, horses ...

- Our EYES remember (smiles, expressions, sceneries, land views, faces, tears ...

- Our EARS remember (insults, whispers, words, poetry, stories, voice tone, music...

- Our NOSE remembers (smells, weather stations, love, people, parents, perfumes...

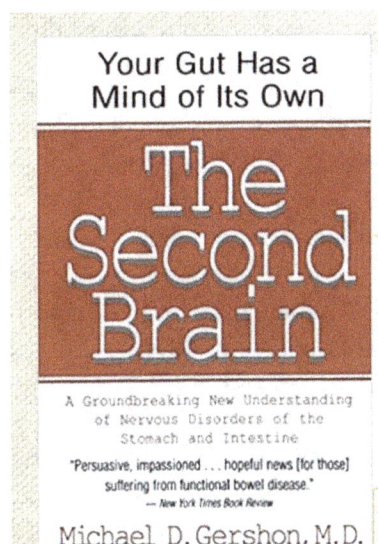

Your Gut Has a Mind of Its Own

The Second Brain

A Groundbreaking New Understanding
of Nervous Disorders of the
Stomach and Intestine

"Persuasive, impassioned . . . hopeful news [for those]
suffering from functional bowel disease."
— *New York Times Book Review*

Michael D. Gershon, M.D.

LUXURIOUS BRAND 2023

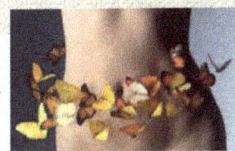

Dopamine & Serotonin

GUT MICROBIOME

- **Care for your gut** microbiome because it contributes to your mental **wellbeing and longevity** through the **SECOND BRAIN** (ENS-Enteric Nervous System). It is nearly as important as your actual brain producing the chemicals to make you **happy** and keep you **healthy.**

Second brain feels INTUITION.
Intuition is inherently a human function.

INTUITION is **a form of intelligence** which is contextual, relational, is holistic, does not have win-loose orientation, goes beyond cause -effect, is beyond conscious mind and archetypal mind.

INTUITION is outstanding for Artists, Entrepreneurs and Researchers and predominant in ♀

Intuition (the 6th sense) and the gut microbiome have been shown to be connected in several ways. Gut microbiome not only affect mood, cognition, and other aspects of brain function, it also influences the immune system, which has been shown to play a role in intuition by allowing us to respond quickly to environmental questions and perceive danger. What will be the relationship with the recently discover brain-immuno-axis is open.

Some people have a heightened sense of intuition or a "gut feeling" that can help them to perceive danger in advance. These responses are not always accurate and can sometimes lead to false alarms or misperceptions. To increase our ability to perceive danger, it is important to stay attuned to our physical and psychological responses, and to be mindful of our surroundings and the information we are receiving through our 5 classical senses but also from our two added senses: Interception and Proprioception.

Humans perceive danger in advance by a combination of physiological and psychological responses. These responses are often triggered by sensory information received through our SEVEN senses (sight, hearing, touch, taste, smell, interception, and proprioception), as well as by other cues such as past experiences, intuition, and environmental context, including people's vibration refer in the EGO chapter.

It is well known the effect of "flying butterflies" in the belly related with our second brain function. It is widely spread that it appears in people in love, nevertheless let me explain you that this is an intuition ring indicating excitement, passion, or fear (stress problems) not really love. True love imply abandonment, confidence, joy, peace; under this circumstance our intuition is not stressed but calm and relax because it is controlled by our oxytocin levels.

The key is to regularly engage in activities and practices that promote feelings of happiness, well-being, and overall contentment, as these are all associated with increased serotonin levels.

When there is an IMBALANCE OF SEROTONIN levels, we can suffer mental and physical health conditions such as:

- Depression: Low levels of serotonin are associated with depression and can contribute to feelings of sadness, hopelessness, and loss of interest in activities, difficulties to sleep. When depressive phenomena are persistent, they are called Dysthymia.
- Anxiety disorders: Imbalances of serotonin can also contribute to symptoms of anxiety, including excessive worry and fear.
- Obsessive-compulsive disorder (OCD): People with OCD may have imbalances in serotonin levels, which can contribute to intrusive thoughts and compulsive behaviors.
- Migraines: Serotonin plays a role in regulating pain, and imbalances of this neurotransmitter can contribute to migraine headaches.
- Irritable bowel syndrome (IBS): Serotonin also helps regulate the contractions of the muscles in the gut. Imbalances of serotonin can contribute to IBS symptoms, such as abdominal pain, bloating, and diarrhea.

The ELECTRIC TRANSCRANEAL STIMULATOR, a magnetic coil applied to the dominant frontal lobe (i.e., right lobe in lefthanded people) for 15 minutes produce after 10-14 sessions an active release of the substances lacking in endogenous depressions (mainly Serotonin and Endorphin). In fact, Israelite children play with electric plugs putting the fingers on it to get an electric discharge; those discharges are anti-depressive, transforming those children into happier ones, and improving their concentration (obviously if they don't get electrocuted for other circumstantial reasons). The advantage of the Electrical transcranial stimulator is that it does not have any side effect or contraindication, but it has another meaning to us, it demonstrates that outside vibrations (see below people's vibrations section) are capable to release and change internal neurotransmitters.

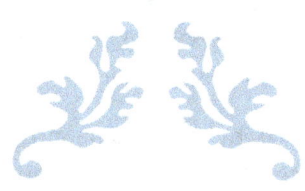

SEROTONIN SYNDROME

We have indicated that Serotonin has broad effects. There are at least 14 different types of serotonin receptors in the brain. Serotonin receptors are divided into seven families (5-HT1 to 5-HT7) based on their structural and functional properties. A brief overview of serotonin receptors and their general functions are listed here to understand the ominous prognosis of a Serotonin Syndrome produced by an overdose.

5-HT1 receptor family, which is primarily involved in the inhibition of adenylate cyclase activity and the regulation of neurotransmitter release

- 5-HT1A: Regulates mood, anxiety, and appetite; it is used with antidepressant drugs.
- 5-HT1B: Modulates mood, cognition, and pain perception; it is used in migraines.
- 5-HT1D: Regulates blood vessel constriction; used in migraines treatment.
- 5-HT1E: Regulating serotonin release and nervous system function.
- 5-HT1F: Regulating pain, migraine, and cerebrovascular tone. Activation can lead to the inhibition of neurotransmitter release, including the release of substance P, a neuropeptide involved in pain sensation. Drugs that activate this receptor can reduce the release of inflammatory peptides involved in migraine pathophysiology.

S-HT2 receptor family, plays important roles in the regulation of many physiological processes and is a target for a variety of therapeutic interventions.
- The 5-HT2A: Regulates mood, perception, and cognition. Located in the central nervous system (CNS) are associated with the Astral-trip effects of psychedelics, such as LSD and psilocybin, and with the therapeutic effects of some antidepressant and anxiolytic drugs.
- The 5-HT2B: Regulates cardiac function and blood pressure, as well certain pathologies, such as pulmonary hypertension and valvular heart disease. It is widely distributed in peripheral tissues, including the heart, lungs, and digestive system.
- The 5-HT2C: Implicated in the regulation of appetite, mood, and addiction. The receptor is expressed both in the brain and in peripheral tissues. Its activation is a potential target for the treatment of obesity, because these receptors can reduce food intake.

The S-HT3 receptor is part of the ligand-gated ion channel superfamily, and they function by allowing the flow of positively charged ions across the cell membrane.
- The 5-HT3: Participates in the regulation of mood, appetite, and nausea. It is present in both central and peripheral nervous systems. Drugs that interact are Ondansetron to prevent nausea and vomiting, and Alosetron to treat irritable bowel syndrome. Some antidepressants and antipsychotics can also interact.

The S-HT4 receptor family have two main subtypes:
- The 5-HT4(a): Regulates the learning and memory and modulate dopamine and acetylcholine release. It is primarily found in the CNS, and used in the treatment of depression and anxiety.
- The 5-HT4(b): Regulates gastrointestinal motility and secretion. It is found in the gastrointestinal tract. It is used in the treatment of irritable bowel syndrome and gastroparesis.

The S-HT5 receptor family located in the brain is not yet understood but play a role in the regulation of dopamine release, cognitive function, and mood.

- The 5-HT5A: Expressed in the hippocampus, a brain region involved in learning and memory. It modulates the release of dopamine in the prefrontal cortex.
- The 5-HT5B: It may regulate mood and anxiety and develop schizophrenia. Its functions are not well characterized.

The S-HT6 receptor participate in learning and memory, as well as in the modulation of mood and behavior. Located in the striatum, cortex, and hippocampus, is involved in cognitive function, motor control, and emotion. It has a role in Alzheimer's disease, Parkinson's disease, schizophrenia, depression, and anxiety.

The S-HT7 receptor regulate mood and cognition, sleep-wake cycle, and cardiovascular functions. It is found in hypothalamus, hippocampus, and cortex, involved in the regulation of emotion, memory, and attention. Its activation can improve cognitive function and promote neuroplasticity. It has a role in depression, anxiety, schizophrenia, and Alzheimer.

Due to the extensive effects of serotonin, an excess of serotonin will produce a risky body disbalance, a SEROTONIN SYNDROME. Serotonin syndrome is a potentially life-threatening episode, can range from mild to severe and develop within hours of taking the serotoninergic substances. The symptoms may include:

- Agitation and restlessness
- Confusion and disorientation
- Rapid heart rate and high blood pressure
- Dilated pupils
- Headache and muscle rigidity
- Tremors and twitching
- Sweating and fever
- Nausea and vomiting
- Seizures and loss of consciousness

In severe cases, it can lead to high fever, muscle rigidity, and organ failure, and dead if not treated promptly. Treatment includes discontinuing the serotonergic substance, providing supportive care, and hospitalization.

Some public figures have been reported to die from serotonin syndrome or at least have been associated with serotonergic substances i.e.

- Philip Seymour Hoffman, an actor, who was found dead in his apartment in 2014 with a mixture of heroin and prescription medications, including a serotonergic antidepressant, in his system.
- Heath Ledger, an actor, who died in 2008 from an accidental overdose of prescription medications, including a serotonergic antidepressant.
- Prince, a musician, who died in 2016 from an accidental overdose of fentanyl, a powerful opioid, but with elevated levels of a serotonergic antidepressant in his system...

In July 2023, the Australia's Therapeutic Goods Administration (TGA) authorized psychiatrists to prescribe MDMA (3,4-methylenedioxymethamphetamine), a synthetic drug that alters mood and perception by binding 2a-receptors but also dopamine receptors; it has been selected for the treatment of post-traumatic stress disorder (PTSD). TGA also authorized

PSILOCYBIN, the active ingredient in magic mushrooms, that stimulate first 2a and after the mystic experience the 1a receptor feeling containment; this is chosen for the treatment-resistant depression.

When overstimulation of the Serotonin systems does not reach the level of the "syndrome", we might be moving at the level of <u>ASTRAL TRIPS</u> if it stimulates 2a-receptors. Already covered in the DMT section, it refers to the concept of leaving one's physical body and exploring our spiritual self, the spiritual or astral realm. These experiences can be either pleasant or unpleasant.

➤ **Pleasant astral trips** may involve feelings of peace, joy, and freedom. The person may encounter beautiful landscapes, positive entities, or have spiritual experiences.
➤ **Unpleasant astral trips** may involve fear, confusion, and negative entities. The person may encounter dark or frightening landscapes and have unpleasant experiences. These trips may result in a feeling of being lost, trapped, or overwhelmed.

Factors that can influence those experiences as pleasant or unpleasant can be:

- Dosage and frequency of the substance responsible for the serotonin overstimulation
- Individual differences in brain chemistry, genetics, and psychological factors
- Environmental factors and surroundings during the experience
- Previous experiences and expectations
- Mental and emotional state of the individual prior to and during the experience.

It's important to note that astral trips are a subjective experience that vary greatly from person to person. Some people may have a mixture of both pleasant and unpleasant experiences. These experiences are not real in a physical sense (although individuals live them as such) but simply manifestation of one's own thoughts and imagination what our Soul had been collecting and keeping. On this regard, they are directly related with the self-understanding, the self-care, the self-growth, and how much our three consciousness have been grown.

In some belief systems, pleasant and unpleasant astral experiences are considered related to concepts of God and Evil. For example, in certain religious or spiritual beliefs, God is seen as a positive and benevolent force, while evil is seen as negative and malevolent. In this context, a pleasant astral trip may involve an encounter with a divine or positive entity, while an unpleasant astral trip may involve an encounter with a negative or evil entity. In any case this is You, what You have collected in your frontal area, the same God that can be good or bad depending on You. This is how we manifest the Infinity Consciousness that we possess.

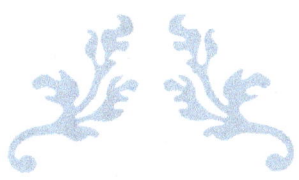

Oxytocin is **the LOVE HORMONE**.

The real life is the only one that allow us to produce **OXYTOCIN** with love, kisses, time spend, nature and sports sharing. This only happens when we are in the PRESENT when we are BEINGs.

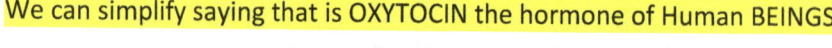

We can simplify saying that is OXYTOCIN the hormone of Human BEINGS

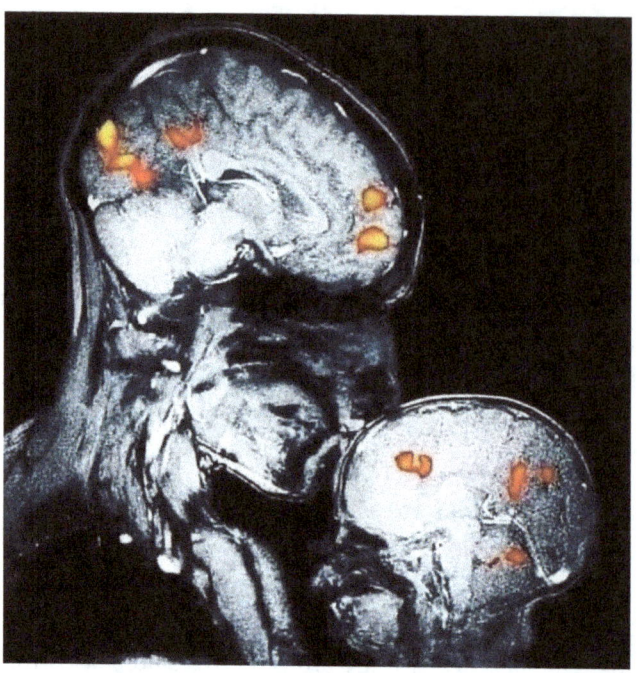

fMRI artificial construction from the below MRI
Why I Captured This MRI of a Mother and Child | Science| Smithsonian Magazine

Oxytocin is often referred to as the "feel-good hormone" or the "love hormone" because of its role in promoting feelings of bonding, trust, and social connection. When people engage in physical touch, such as hugging or cuddling, the nerve impulses are sent from sensory receptors in the skin to *the hypothalamus*, triggering the release of oxytocin. This release of oxytocin then circulates in the bloodstream and interacts with oxytocin receptors in various parts of the body, producing its effects.

SOCIAL SUPPORT. Humans are good in social support. It requires emotional bonding that starts in mother-baby and goes on during all our life. Start in the Prefrontal Cortex (PFC) and go to the amygdala (where the emotions reside) lowering stress hormones. In some interactions such the ones of CARE-GIVING it goes to the reward pattern and stimulates EPOs reducing even more stress hormones. It provides positive emotions, greater reward activation and increase Serotonin.

Oxytocin receptors are found in the brain, the uterus, the heart, and the blood vessels. In the brain, are found in several regions involved in regulation of mood, emotions, and social behavior, such as the *hypothalamus, amygdala, and prefrontal cortex.* In the uterus, oxytocin receptors play a crucial role in labor and delivery, as they are involved in the contraction of the uterus during childbirth. Oxytocin receptors in the heart and blood vessels are involved in regulation of blood pressure, as well as in the formation of social bonds and the promotion of feelings of love and affection. Overall, the distribution of oxytocin receptors throughout the body helps to ensure that the hormone is able to produce its wide-ranging effects, from regulation of labor and child delivery to regulation of mood, emotions, and social behavior.

In addition to its effects is also involved in a range of physiological processes, including pain, digestion, and blood pressure regulation. This release of oxytocin is associated with increased feelings of happiness, trust, and relaxation, and can help to reduce feelings of stress and anxiety. Its effects on PAIN REGULATION are important. It can reduce sensitivity to pain and can also relieve chronic pain conditions such as headaches and menstrual cramps. Furthermore since oxytocin is the bonding hormone any detachment from bonding (i.e. Social Rejection, Lover detachment...) activates pain brain centers.

In terms of brain structure and function, women may have a greater number of oxytocin receptors in certain brain regions compared to men; nevertheless, as we will see below the Nudity Processing system mediated by Oxytocin is twice as big in men.

➢ In women, oxytocin have a great impact on social cognition, social bonding, and maternal behavior related with the hormones of the *hypothalamus*, the emotions of the *amygdala* and the empathy and social recognition in the *cingulate cortex*.
➢ In men, oxytocin has been associated with increased trust and prosocial behavior, as well as increased sexual behavior because can increase testosterone and aggression not clearly understood. Being a hormone linked to social behaviors and emotions, some research suggests that may play a role in JEALOUSY in romantic relationships particularly in men.

Jealousy is a complex emotion involving multiple neurotransmitters such as:

- Serotonin: Low levels of serotonin have been associated with increased jealousy and possessiveness.
- Dopamine: Increased dopamine levels in response to a perceived threat to a romantic relationship may contribute to feelings of jealousy.
- Norepinephrine: High levels of norepinephrine have been associated with feelings of jealousy, particularly in response to a threat to a relationship.
- Oxytocin: May play a role particularly in romantic relationships.

The increase of Oxytocin in women appears in:

- Ovulation: Oxytocin levels tend to increase around the time of ovulation, which is when a woman's ovaries release an egg.
- Pregnancy: During pregnancy, oxytocin levels increase in response to the growing fetus, which stimulates the uterus. Oxytocin is also involved in the onset of labor and helps to regulate the intensity and duration of contractions during childbirth.
- Breastfeeding: Oxytocin levels increase when a woman is breastfeeding, which helps to stimulate milk production and facilitate the bonding between mother and baby.
- Sexual arousal: Oxytocin levels also increase during sexual arousal and orgasm in women, which can enhance sexual pleasure and facilitate bonding with a sexual partner.

The increase of Oxytocin in men appears in:

- Sexual arousal and orgasm: Oxytocin levels have been found to increase in men during sexual arousal and orgasm, which can enhance sexual pleasure and facilitate bonding with a sexual partner.
- Parental bonding: Some studies have suggested that oxytocin levels may increase in men during parental bonding with a child, such as during skin-to-skin contact or when playing with a child.
- Social bonding: Oxytocin has also been linked to social bonding in men, with some studies suggesting that it can increase trust and prosocial behavior.
- Brain has its own <u>Nudity Processing system</u> sexually dimorphic, twice as big in males. It starts in the occipito-temporal lobe. This area fires the insular, *amygdala* (the Bed Nucleus of the Stria Terminalis-BST) and then the medial preoptic area (MPOA) of the *hypothalamus* to initiate male sexual behavior. The MPOA activates the paraventricular nucleus of *hypothalamus* (PVN) to release OXYTOCIN into the cerebrospinal fluid (CSF) and into the blood system via the Pituitary. Since the CSF is renewed every 6 hours the physiological effect in man can last for 6 hours. Noticed that when oxytocin is injected into the spinal fluid in rats, erection occurs.
- Stress reduction: Oxytocin can help to reduce stress and anxiety in men and may increase during periods of relaxation and stress reduction.

To build an oxytocin-rich life, you can consider the following:

1. <u>Connect with others</u>: Oxytocin is released in the brain during social interactions, such as hugs, touch, and intimate conversations. Make time for meaningful relationships with friends and family and seek out opportunities to connect with others.
2. Exercise: Regular physical activity has been shown to increase oxytocin levels, particularly when performed in groups or with a partner. Consider joining a team sport, taking group fitness classes, or going for a walk or run with a friend.
3. Practice mindfulness: Mindfulness practices, such as meditation and yoga, have been shown to increase oxytocin levels and improve well-being. Incorporate mindfulness into your daily routine to help reduce stress and promote feelings of calm and connection.
4. <u>Volunteer</u>: Giving back to others has been shown to increase oxytocin levels and boost feelings of happiness and fulfillment. Consider volunteering your time and skills to support a cause or community organization that is important to you.
5. <u>Show gratitude</u>: Expressing gratitude and focusing on the things in your life that you are thankful for can increase oxytocin levels and improve well-being. Consider keeping a gratitude journal, writing thank-you notes, or simply taking time each day to reflect on the things you are grateful for.

The key is to regularly get engaged in activities and practices that promote feelings of connection, trust, and well-being, as these are all associated with increased oxytocin levels.

And remember that HAPPINESS affect the behavior of others, spread in social networks, is infective because it activates our Mirrow Neurons as we will se later on, creating PERSONAL SYNCHRONIZATION and empathy.

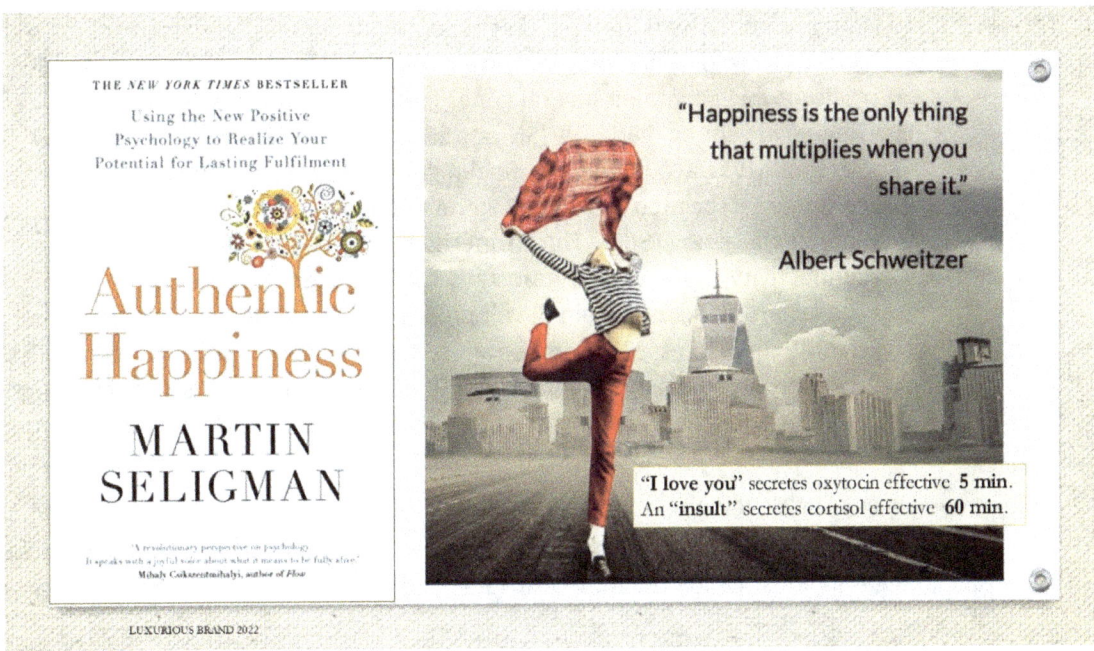

THE *NEW YORK TIMES* BESTSELLER

Using the New Positive
Psychology to Realize Your
Potential for Lasting Fulfilment

Authentic
Happiness

MARTIN
SELIGMAN

'A revolutionary perspective on psychology.
It speaks with a joyful voice about what it means to be fully alive.'
Mihaly Csikszentmihalyi, author of *Flow*

LUXURIOUS BRAND 2022

"Happiness is the only thing
that multiplies when you
share it."

Albert Schweitzer

"I love you" secretes oxytocin effective **5 min.**
An "insult" secretes cortisol effective **60 min.**

Oxytocin imbalances have been implicated in various psychological and psychiatric disorders, including autism, social anxiety disorder, borderline personality disorder, post-traumatic stress disorder (PTSD), schizophrenia, and depression.

Low levels of oxytocin have been associated with increased risk of suicide and suicidal behavior, although suicide is a complex issue with many potential contributing factors, including mental health disorders, stress, trauma, and access to lethal means. Noticed that in countries where assisted suicide is allowed, people with post-traumatic stress disorder (PTSD), schizophrenia, and depression have the risk to ask for it.

In spite to the fact that autism **spectrum disorder (ASD)** is characterized by changes in communication and social interaction in where the Mirrow Neurons are implicated (see below), the main cause is changes in brain development and function by combination of genetic and environmental factors that affect behavior. Changes associated with autism are:

1. Altered Neural Connectivity: Individuals with autism may exhibit differences in the way brain cells communicate and form connections, potentially affecting regions of the brain involved in social interaction, communication, and sensory processing.
2. Abnormal Brain Growth: There may be differences in the size and patterns of brain growth, especially during early childhood. These abnormalities can impact brain organization and function.
3. Mirror Neurons: Mirror neurons are a type of brain cells that are involved in imitation, empathy, and understanding the actions and intentions of others. Dysfunction of mirror neurons may contribute to the social and communication difficulties observed in individuals with autism.
4. Genetic Factors: There are mutations and genetic variations associated with autism.
    a. Mutations in specific genes: Such as the **oxytocin receptor gene** (OXTR), the N-methyl-D-aspartate receptor-related protein gene (NMDAR), which is a **glutamate receptor**, and the nerve growth factor gene (NGF), among others.
    b. Mutations in synapse-related genes: Mutations in genes related to synaptic function, such as the SHANK3 gene, NLGN3 gene, and NRXN1 gene. These genes play a crucial role in communication and connectivity between brain cells.

c. Copy number variations (CNVs): Some individuals with autism may have duplications or deletions in certain regions of DNA, such as the 15q11-13 region, which contains several genes involved in brain development.

d. Single nucleotide variants (SNVs): SNVs are changes in a single DNA base. Several SNVs have been identified in genes associated with autism, such as the contactin-associated protein 2 gene (CNTNAP2) and the tuberous sclerosis complex 2 gene (TSC2). The former is involved in neuronal development and connectivity, particularly important for language and social communication. The latter is linked to brain development and function.

5. Environmental Influences: Environmental factors, such as prenatal complications, exposure to certain substances, and early life experiences, can also contribute to the development of autism. However, specific environmental factors and their interactions with genetic factors are still being studied.

These changes in brain development and function are not unique to autism and may also be seen in other neurodevelopmental disorders. Further research is needed to fully understand the brain changes in autism and how they contribute to the development of the disorder.

Now that you know the function of Neurotransmitters and understand the Dopamine Play, it is it is time to analyze MANIPULATION.

➢ From the manipulator point of view: dopamine may be involved in the satisfaction when they successfully manipulate someone. Serotonin, which is associated with mood and social behavior, may play a role in the emotional manipulation of others. And oxytocin, which is often referred to as the "bonding hormone," may be involved in the creation of strong social bonds that are exploited in manipulation. All those play a role in Cultural Conditioning, in the pleasure of political sympathies or in the ambition of power. The process of manipulation obviously involves many factors, including environmental and psychological factors, together with the complex interplay of neurotransmitters.

➢ The individuals being manipulated with tactics of flattery and promises of rewards, experience an increase in dopamine. Using threats or other forms of negative reinforcement, decrease serotonin levels, and result in feelings of depression or anxiety. Not only the tactics can influence but the individual's underlying psychological and physical health, and the context in which the manipulation occurs.

Among the threats and negative reinforcement, we have:

• Physical violence: The threat of physical harm or actual physical violence to intimidate or control someone, can lead to feelings of fear and anxiety, which are associated with an increase in the release of cortisol.

• Verbal abuse: Insults, name-calling, and other forms of verbal abuse to make them more susceptible to manipulation, lead to feelings of anxiety and depression, which are associated with changes in the levels of serotonin and norepinephrine.

• Emotional manipulation: Guilt or shame to feel responsible or by suggesting that they will be punished if they don't comply is similar to verbal abuse.

• Blackmail: using sensitive or embarrassing information to blackmail someone into doing what they want, produce a range of emotional responses, including confusion and self-doubt, associated with changes in levels of dopamine, serotonin, and cortisol.

- Withholding rewards or affection: such as money or gifts, can be associated with changes in levels of dopamine, in the circuit of reward and motivation.
- Gaslighting: A manipulator may try to make someone doubt their own perceptions or memories, in order to gain control over them. It influences are similar to blackmail.
- Social isolation: from their support system, such as by discouraging them from spending time with friends or family, in order to make them more dependent on the manipulator, behave similarly to verbal abuse or emotional manipulation.

The effects of negative reinforcement tactics depend on individual factors, including genetics, personality traits, and previous life experiences. And when persisting in time they develop CHRONIC STRESS with anxiety, depression and suicide.

To recognize those tactics and their potential to manipulate and control behavior, allow us to resist and help individuals to protect themselves maintaining their autonomy and free will.

> To overcome life difficulties (monetary, social, personal) shape our consciousness.

MONEY SCRIPTS

Money scripts are unconscious beliefs and attitudes that individuals have towards money and wealth, which influence their financial behaviors and decisions. These scripts can come from a variety of sources, including family, friends, media, and personal experiences.

This is just an example of how close your <u>unconscious mind</u> is acting on you. It is worth mentioning due to the widespread problem of stress linked to money lack or abundance. It's important to be aware of one's money scripts and how they may be contributing to financial stress, and to work on developing healthy and positive beliefs and habits around money. This can include setting financial goals, creating a budget, seeking professional advice, and practicing mindfulness and self-care.

> Our relationship with **MONEY is the first cause of STRESS** in the Occidental world.
>
> Stress interferes in our accurate judgement, consequently, decisions on money issues are particularly inaccurate.

Ironically more money does not solve our problems or release our stress. And there is NO predictable correlation between money and happiness. <u>Happiness</u> is, on the contrary, related with <u>strong</u> <u>personal</u> <u>relationships and the self-sense of accomplishment</u>. In other words, the question is not making more money but instead developing better and healthier relationship with it.

> ➤ **Money-related disorders** are patterns of self-complex behavior related with financial habits. They are the result of distorted beliefs about money that we have grown up with. Childhood interpretations of familiar financial flashpoint events build our believes about money. Financial problems are so painful, stressful, and dramatic that they mark our lives, lasting and worsen with adulthood. They are like movie-scripts. The "Money-Scripts", buried in our animal brain, are unconsciously used as "interpreter mechanisms" to overgeneralized behaviors, shaping the way we think and interact with money as adults.

> ➤ **Principles of healthy finances** are extraordinary simple and limited. Only four issues are essential:

>> 1.- Save now and invest for the future.

>> 2.- Spend reasonably to be able to enjoy life and achieve your goals.

>> 3.- Always spend less than you earn

>> 4.- Beware of investments that seem too good to be true, because they probably are.

Everything should be predictable, but unfortunately it gets triggered by the Stress and Anxiety linked to our early money experiences. As a result, and despite the simplicity, most of us have, to some extent, financial unhealthy situations leading to **3 categories of money disorders** from slight to severe:

1.- **Money avoidance** (includes **excessive risk aversion**) in the two versions

-**Financial denial**: When instead of facing our financial reality, we minimize any financial problem and refuse to think about it. i.e., avoiding looking at our bank account or credit card bill.

- **Financial rejection**: When we feel guilt accumulating money -regardless of the amount-

2.- <u>**Worship of money**</u> (includes **gambling** problems, **work-alcoholism** for money, and **excessive spending**). Money ambition brings people far, but could detach them from their family and their reality:

- **Hoarding**: When hoarding objects or money provides a sense of security and relief.

- **Compulsive buying**: Compulsive buyers do not know how to correctly handle the concern that money exerts on them. It is a behavior learned in childhood, in which they were taught that shopping provides a temporary escape from the feeling of worry and anxiety. Thanks to dopamine these people think and anticipate the pleasure they will feel when they buy, but it is momentary, and ended causing anxiety.

3.- <u>**Money and personal relationships**</u>: (including **financial dependency**, classical of women):

- **Financial infidelity**: that is to say "little lies" about our expenses or the way we handle our finances to a family member or a partner. i.e., when you agreed on a budget to buy something, but then you exceed it, and you prefer to lie before accepting that you did not respect the agreement. There are extreme examples like taking out a second mortgage on the sly or opening a secret bank account.

- **Waste**: it is when you give money to others regardless of whether you are financially solvent or not, having problems refusing to lend money, sacrificing your own financial well-being for the good of others. A common example is when parents continue to help financially their adult children, who should be able to support themselves. This disorder becomes more common when there are economic crises or when there is a feeling of guilt for family members who are less fortunate financially.

Almost everyone has problems with money linked to Money-Scripts learn when childhood, unless the problem is identified and solved during adult time, or the child is trained specifically on healthy finances.

In my case and in spite that I can properly council third people in consultancy, I, myself am under the "Waste problem" sacrificing my own financial wellbeing because it makes me happy when I am able to expend money in others and trying to find money desperately in periods of contracted finances, despite my slight "Money avoidance".

➤ **The basics of financial health** are not complicated, and we are all capable of mastering them regardless of our level of wealth:

<u>The first</u> thing is **to identify** and accept we suffer from a money disorder, having in mind that all of us are highly resistant to change.

<u>The second</u> step is to challenge our distorted beliefs and put into practice healthy financial habits.

All these make us materially richer, emotionally richer and relieve the stress link to money.

Obviously, neurotransmitters play a role in regulating emotions and behaviors related to money. The ones associated with money and financial behavior are mainly:

- Serotonin: Low levels of serotonin are linked to impulsive <u>risk-taking</u> financial behaviors. If you are this way try to find a Serotonin Life.
- Dopamine: Associated with the pleasure and reward systems of the brain has been linked to <u>overspending</u> and compulsive buying.
- Norepinephrine: This neurotransmitter is related to stress and arousal, and high levels have been associated with <u>financial anxiety</u> and stress.
- GABA: GABA is a neurotransmitter that helps to regulate anxiety and stress. Low levels of GABA have been linked to increased anxiety and <u>worry about money</u>.

As already stated in the chapter of neurotransmitters

<mark>We are what our neurotransmitters let us to be.</mark>

Although simultaneously we learn that we are a Trinity close to God or in God. That our Mind-Body-Soul is capable to change brain dynamics and chemistry, advise and guide, live with us, prepared life for miracles, build and create the world.

Controlling money disorders that are linked to the unconscious mind can be challenging, but it's possible with the right approach. Here are some strategies that can help:

1. <u>Identify unconscious beliefs</u> and attitudes: Awareness is the first step in changing unconscious money scripts. Write down your thoughts and feelings about money and look for patterns and themes that may be contributing to your financial behaviors.
2. Challenge negative beliefs: Once you have identified negative or limiting money scripts, it's important to challenge and reframe them. This can involve questioning the evidence for these beliefs and replacing them with more positive and empowering beliefs about money.
3. Practice mindfulness: Mindfulness practices, such as meditation, can help individuals become more aware of their thoughts and feelings, and can increase their ability to control negative or automatic thoughts.
4. Seek professional help: A financial therapist or psychologist can help individuals gain insight into their unconscious beliefs and provide strategies for changing negative financial behaviors.
5. Surround yourself with <u>positive influences</u>: Surrounding yourself with people who have positive and healthy attitudes towards money can help to counteract negative money scripts and reinforce positive financial behaviors. This also will be related with the importance of the topic of next chapter, the mirror neurons.
6. Engage in <u>positive financial behaviors</u>: Engaging in positive financial behaviors, such as saving, investing, and budgeting, can help individuals build self-esteem and confidence in their ability to manage money.

It's important to remember that changing unconscious money scripts takes time and effort, but the benefits of overcoming negative financial behaviors can have a significant impact on financial health and overall well-being.

Do not close yourself, go to be free, be part of the solution-seeking generation. **The best things in life are for FREE** but they are also transient and fleeting, while the second good things in life are very expensive. Furthermore, the best things in life cannot be collected with money because **<u>do not belong to us</u>**, therefore it is essential to be grateful for what we receive. The years after COVID, are where all of us are going to learn what is important. Regardless cars, houses, richness, we will turn to basic things: nature, sun, family, people that care, healthy food. Next years will be to balance senses of pleasure and authenticity of love.

To be useful to help others, we must think first in ourselves; it is like in aircraft's depressurization: Put your mask on before you try to help others. It is a year of serendipity and miracles. Be prepared.

"In life you have to avoid three geometric figures: vicious circles, love triangles and the square minds" Mario Benedetti

"Happiness is internal, not external, therefore, it does not depend on what we have, but on what we are" Pablo Neruda

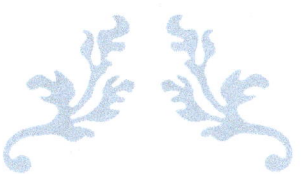

MIRROR NEURONS

Mirror neurons are a type of brain cell that are activated both when an individual performs a certain action and when they observe someone else perform the same action. Mirror neurons are primarily found in the brain's premotor cortex and the inferior parietal cortex, specifically in areas known as *the inferior frontal gyrus* (IFG) and the *inferior parietal lobule* (IPL). These regions are involved in motor planning and execution, as well as in understanding and interpreting the actions and intentions of others.

Mirror neurons are thought to play a critical role in social cognition and empathy. By allowing us to understand and imitate the actions and emotions of others, they help us to understand and respond to the behavior of others, and to learn new skills through observation. They also play a role in the development of language, as they allow us to understand the meaning of words and sentences by simulating the actions and emotions they describe.

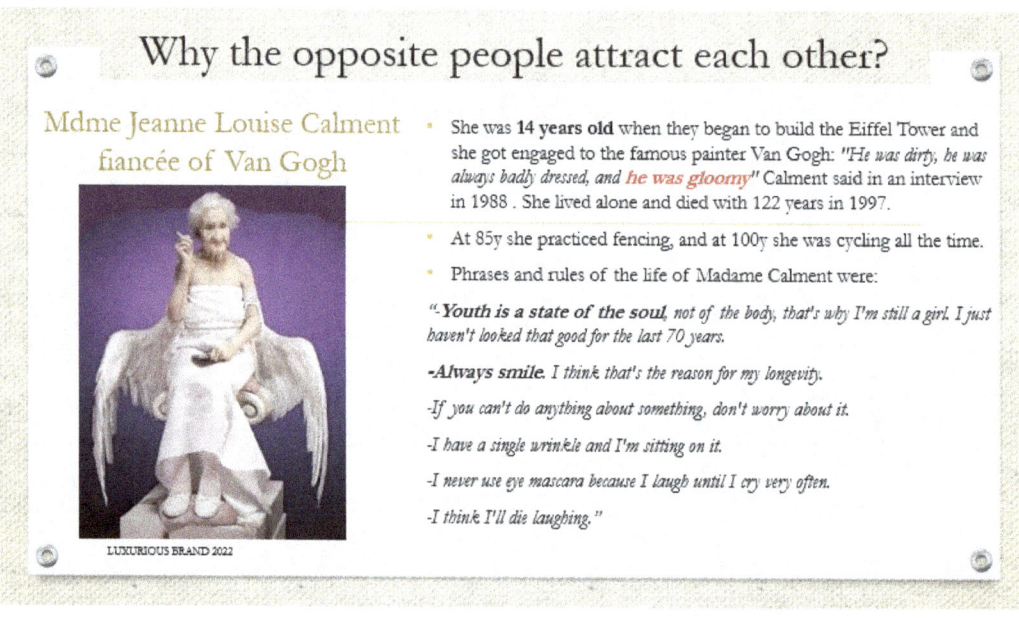

A nice story of Mirror Neurons working in complementary people.

Mirrow neurons take visual, auditory and tactile information track the emotional information and activate our amygdala (where emotions reside) in order to feel the same emotion.

Its role in acting, marketing, and any convincing arts is essential. Uploading selected pictures to IG is a way to stimulate your friends' mirror neurons. Mirror neurons are the ones that explain why we feel that **we "know" movie stars** and TV personalities and why we **unconsciously bond with actors**, artists, and speakers (*) we see on screens or on stage. Everyone can stimulate reflex behavior (**mimetics** i.e., to yawn or to learn by doing), some people can stimulate **empathy**, but it is not easy to develop true **intuition** about someone; only people with a solid spiritual foundation (and "some" people *in love*) are able to do so.

Uploading selected pictures to IG is a way to stimulate your friends' mirror neurons. Mirror neurons are the ones that explain why we feel that **we "know" movie stars** and TV personalities and why we **unconsciously bond with actors**, artists, and speakers (*) we see on screens or on stage. Everyone can stimulate reflex behavior (**mimetics** i.e., to yawn or to learn by doing), some people can stimulate **empathy**, but it is not easy to develop true **intuition** about someone; only people with a solid spiritual foundation (and "some" people *in love*) are able to do so.

(*) Noticed that it also happens to speakers (teachers), as well as mentors. The bond with University professors is also well known; I am acquainted with the feeling of being watched, admired, followed, trusted and relay upon.

(**) This is believed by "all" people *in love* and makes them to think that the lover has changed when does not behave as expected.

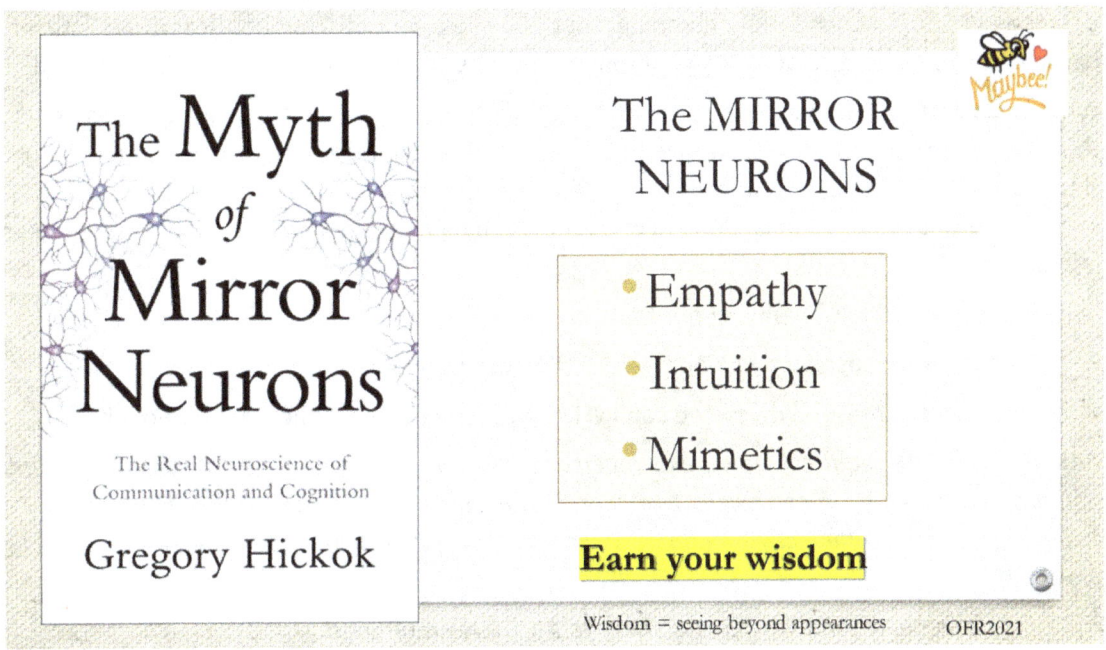

They are the essential part of our spiritual layer. MIRROR NEURONS are a Group of Neurons dedicated **to understanding the intention of others**.

They guide and direct 3 main behaviors.

1. EMPATHY
2. INTUITION
3. MIMETICS

Understanding and be *in love* is a question either of EMPAHTY or INTUITION

IF PEOPLE ARE EQUAL	The bond is based on **INTUITION** that allow you to understand and pre-judge the other person feelings and activities and to enhance your admiration towards them.
IF THEY ARE COMPLEMENTARY	The role of **EMPATHY** helps to feel sensitive to the lack of the other person, understanding and helping them, admiring and bonding with them on the effort. This is why opposite people get in love.

INTUITION GUIDES YOU

Mirror neurons as the intuition, **ignite BEFORE** the action takes place, indicating that WE KNEW before it happens, that we are SPIRITUAL beings capable to feel and understand BEFORE it happens. That our knowledge and spirituality is guided as gods and goddesses **BEFORE things happen.**

To fire those neurons, <mark>we need a MIRROR</mark> … How much distant this mirror can be, depend on you. It depends on how much trained you are, how much spiritual you are, and how much sensitive you can be.

But the MIRROR is essential, meaning that as soon you disconnect from this mirror, particularly if he-she-it is far away, your mirror neurons and your intuition get disconnected.

What this means is that you must get connected with the subject even @ distance, to assure that the subject of your interested will be influenced by your empathy or by your intuition. Happily enough, now a days Internet, YouTube, Instagram, movies etc. allow the function of mirror neurons. Part of this influence is known by politician and TV to extend his/her influences.

- That is **the reason why** → our DEAMS come true.
- This is **the reason why** → our INTUITION from others exists.
- This is **the reason why** → we can INFLUENCE others if we concentrate enough.

*Although the time required could be as much as 20 years (**average time** necessary to assure a political change as soon as you start to change the thinking of the society) We still are quite imperfect! Unless influence is enhanced with fear (as the Nazis' propaganda or gender violence).*

- This is **the reason why** → we arrive to AN IDEA simultaneously with many others.

Providing that it is a business idea, it must be put into practice as soon as possible to succeed, before the rest of the people also will do it. Is part of the concept of the OPPORTUNITY WINDOW.

World is connected throughout by our mirror neurons. (now-a-days facilitated by Internet)

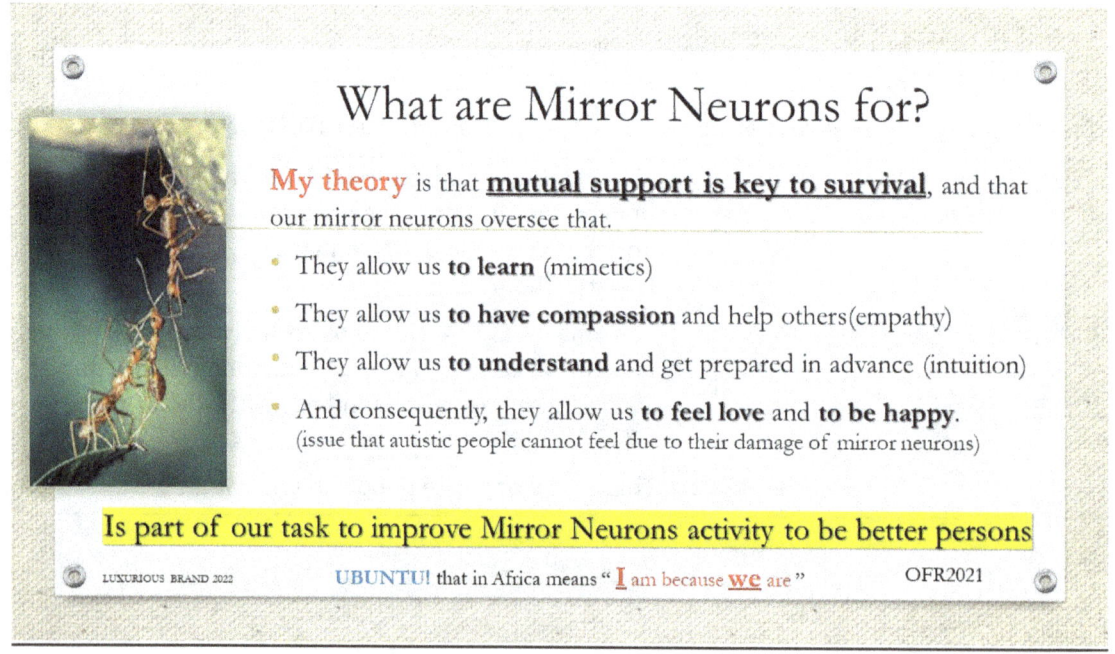

What are Mirror Neurons for?

My theory is that **mutual support is key to survival**, and that our mirror neurons oversee that.

- They allow us **to learn** (mimetics)
- They allow us **to have compassion** and help others(empathy)
- They allow us **to understand** and get prepared in advance (intuition)
- And consequently, they allow us **to feel love** and **to be happy**. (issue that autistic people cannot feel due to their damage of mirror neurons)

<mark>Is part of our task to improve Mirror Neurons activity to be better persons</mark>

LUXURIOUS BRAND 2022   UBUNTU! that in Africa means " I am because we are "   OFR2021

> By improving the life of other you improve your own life.

Unfortunately, according to Thorstein Veblen

"The tendency to altruism plays a secondary role in our society, since the class that ends up **excelling**, *is the one he called* **"leisure class"** *and does so by virtue of* **selfish** *attitudes."* (Trump is an example).

After seen the movie of "The Secret" (a 2006 Australian-American spirituality documentary consisting of a series of interviews") you understand how powerful rising dreams can be. We create the future in this way. We are human BEings. REALITY is an eternal PRESENT. We only can "BE" here & now.

WHAT IS MARKETING DOING? STIMULATING MIRROR NEURONS.

- ❑ If an influencer sees it attractive, they Will see it attractive.
- ❑ If an influencer shows it nicely, they Will find it nice.
- ❑ I an influencer smiles, they Will smile. (if you do not smile, they will be suspicious)
- ❑ If an influencer is convincing, they Will be convinced.
- ❑ If an influencer thinks of it, they Will think on it.

Be GOOD in marketing means that your MIRROR NEURONS are well trained.

Our intuition arrives so far that modify our body even without knowing it, and sometimes we can see and measure it. That is the case of the **Psychological Forcing**, a fundamental concept in magic, versus **Free Will**. If we have been manipulated by the language, time and/or gaze of a magician, one second after to choose what we have been inducted or forced to do, our pupil dilates 4 times the original size. Meaning that our body knows in advance when we have been manipulated. Indicating as in the case of hypnosis an arousal or susceptibility. These are changes of the autonomic nervous system controlled by the unconscious mind. The sympathetic nervous system is responsible for the "fight or flight" response, which leads to pupil dilation which allows more light to enter the eye and improves visual acuity in low-light conditions. The parasympathetic nervous system, on the other hand, promotes relaxation and slows down the body's processes, which can result in pupil contraction. It's like saying if you keep your attention focused on your opinion you contract your pupil if you surrender to an external influence, the magician's influence, you dilate it.

Our HIGH LEVEL CONCIOUSNESS (the one described in the multilayered body chapter) is Intuitive and therefore is contextual, relational, holistic, without the win-lose orientation, beyond the cause-effect and beyond conscious and archetypal mind, it is a superior intelligence.

In the chapter of Serotonin life, we located our own personal intuition in the Second Brain, the ENS or Enteric Nervous System in the Dopamine-Serotonin system of the intestine.

The prelude to consider something as individual conscious begins with a **Brain unconscious register** that will be used to modify the activity when it becomes conscious, it is the so called first Wave Stimulus. Our unconscious brain registers can modify everything in advance, the so-called **Efferent Copy** responding in advance to the first wave.

An example is the Saccadic suppression: Our eyes are permanently moving jumping from one side to other of an image or a book, this abrupt or saccadic movements are 3 times per second. Under these circumstances we will not be able to focus or see a static image, to correct this our brain that know it in advance create a Saccadic suppression, in which the brain temporarily suppresses visual information during eye movements to avoid double vision.

Another example is that we are permanently talking with ourselves, but we recognize it as our own softly speaking voice. In schizophrenia nevertheless, people recognize his internal voice as external, laud and strange. In telepathy we intuitively hear the internal softly voice of the other person. We know that this voice is soft or laud controlling the size of the brain waves of the auditive cortex.

Brain is not always able to control everything, in fact the dreams built by our subconscious mind cannot be controlled, they are somehow independent although we read in the Hypnosis Chapters that Lucid Dreams can be partially controlled.

If the Brain do not act properly during the pre-informing process through its Efferent Copy, he will find an explanation confabulating a story to justify the way of acting in the conscious phase, as we explained previously.

To create a conscious action, we need a Second Wave stimulus producing a massive response in the whole brain. If the response of the second stimulus is too ordered or too chaotic it remains unconscious. If it is slightly incoherent and go through the Thalamus, the action become conscious.

<mark>The Thalamus is an essential hub to bring an action conscious.</mark>

But bear in mind that the Second Wave that will bring the stimulus in your conscious life, is produced by a massive response of the whole brain. Therefore, could be far from the original stimulus that produced the First Wave in the unconscious brain.

Therefore, we are the ones that build our Conscious Life, our Reality, we are the creators of our World. Do not be surprised when the reality of your unconscious memory (as in the Astral trips) is different, is magical, is universal, is without limits, is without space, is a miracle.

INTUITION is a feeling or thought to guide you. It helps to make a decision or comprehend something. It is a subconscious process taking into account experiences, memories, and pattern recognition.

PREMONITION, on the other hand, is a feeling or belief about the future. It is often in the form of a foreboding or ominous sensation. Initially taken as paranormal or supernatural it is obvious that as much as we know, more natural is considered.

Some theories suggest that premonitions may be related to the body's fight-or-flight response, which is a physiological reaction to perceived threats that prepares the body for immediate action. In this scenario, the body may release stress hormones and trigger physical changes, such as increased heart rate and heightened senses, in response to a premonition. Others believe that premonitions may be related to unconscious awareness of subtle cues or stimuli that are not consciously perceived, such as changes in body language or tone of voice. In this scenario, the body may react to these stimuli even if the individual is not consciously aware of them.

In the case of <u>premonitions dreams</u>, our visual cortex gets involved. The topic of premonition dreams is still highly debated and falls within the realm of parapsychology, which explores phenomena beyond the scope of mainstream scientific understanding.

- One theory that has been suggested is the concept of **precognition**, which posits that certain individuals may have the ability to access information about future events through **extrasensory perception (ESP)**. This theory suggests that premonition dreams could be a manifestation of this precognitive ability, allowing individuals to foresee events before they happen. It may involve the ability to access information beyond the spacetime constrains and as such involve non-local or non-linear aspects of consciousness and entering into the quantum physics, as in case of telepathy.
- One explanation is the **chance or coincidence**. This means that the dream may seem to predict the future event, but it is simply a random occurrence and not actually related to the event.
- Another explanation is that may be related to **unconscious processing of information**. For example, an individual may have encountered information about a future event during their waking life, and this information may be processed and incorporated into their dream.

Let me explain you a premonition event that I lived in first person: *In my twenties I was travelling to Palenque in Mexico in a civil aircraft of few passengers. The suitcases did not arrived and I was worried thinking that we have lost everything while living in the middle of the forest. In spite of the luxurious camp that night I slept badly. I dreamed that my house in Barcelona was burning (fire came from the store of the ground floor), that the glasses of skylights in the yard were blown, and that trying to escape through a narrow corridor I fell down to the burning flat. Next morning, I was in shock and I explained with detail my dream to my mom; both agreed to linked the dream with the luggage problem and we were convinced that it was definitively lost. Surprisingly, our suitcases arrived one day latter, and although worried by my vivid dream there were no further problems in the trip.*

Coming back home around two months later (my memories are loose) we went to the winter opening day of Barcelona Liceo Opera-house at night. After going to sleep we get up around 4:00 with the house burning from the ground store. We lost everything, things happens as I had dreamed except that I took care not to felt down in the corridor.

Constructions in Palenque in Mexico and Tikal in Guatemala are considered to capture Telluric Forces by an interaction between the Earth's magnetic field that can impact living beings. As in the Astral trips-shamanic rituals (scientifically explained in the chapter of Neurotransmitters), the Telluric Forces claim to connect the individual to the subtlety of nature, the intangible, the Force.

Scientific understanding of the world is constantly evolving, and although the Earth's magnetic field can interact with structures, it is very small and not easily noticeable. In some cases, such as with large metal structures like bridges or buildings with extensive metal components, the interaction may be stronger. Nevertheless, the term of "telluric forces" is an archeoastronomy term to describe the influence of the Earth's magnetic field on the orientation and design of ancient monuments and structures to align them with astronomical events that express cultural and religious beliefs, and it is not scientifically proved up to now.

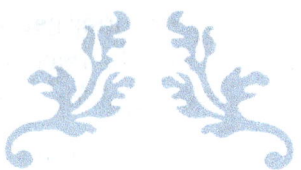

THE VERB

At the beginning it was The WORD, and the word was GOD..., St. Jones said in the BIBLE.

We will dedicate this chapter to closely understand that thanks to the WORD we are GOD or close to GOD. And that WORD introduced in the Bible only belong to the Human species in its elaborate way. Thanks to the WORD we have been able to create, to understand, to build, to transform... to act as a GOD in our world and we are still improving to the level of LIBERATION to the level of to understand and fully function with our Trinity (Mind-Body-Soul).

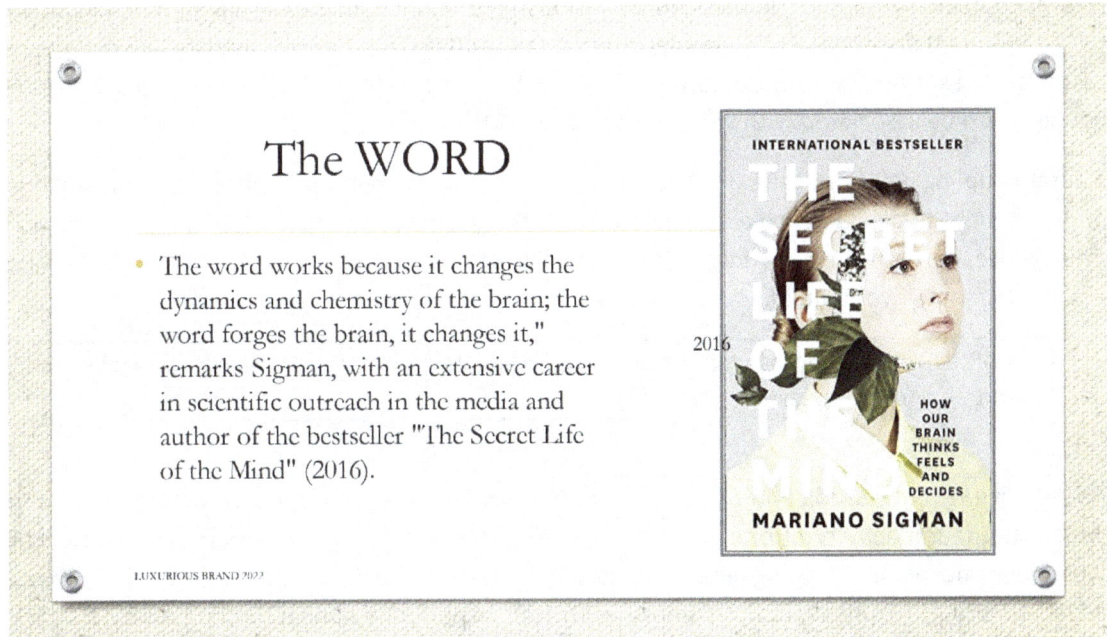

The WORD

- The word works because it changes the dynamics and chemistry of the brain; the word forges the brain, it changes it," remarks Sigman, with an extensive career in scientific outreach in the media and author of the bestseller "The Secret Life of the Mind" (2016).

LUXURIOUS BRAND 2022

INTERNATIONAL BESTSELLER
THE SECRET LIFE OF THE MIND
2016
HOW OUR BRAIN THINKS FEELS AND DECIDES
MARIANO SIGMAN

SPOKEN LANGUAGE

SPOKEN LANGUAGE has a significant impact on brain chemistry and dynamics. When we hear spoken language, processing sounds, meanings, emotions, and context regions are activated and can lead to changes in brain chemistry and dynamics, such as the release of neurotransmitters and the strengthening of neural connections. This is essential to shape Human Consciousness.

The effect in brain of storytelling include.

> 1. **NEURAL COUPLING**. A story activates parts in the brain that allows the listener to turn the story into their own ideas and experiences thanks to the process called neural coupling.

Neural coupling refers to the synchronization or coordination of neural activity between different brain regions. It refers to the idea that different parts of the brain work together in a coordinated manner to perform various tasks and to process information. Neural coupling can occur at different levels of the brain, from local interactions between neurons within a brain region, to long-range interactions between brain regions that are located far apart from each other.

Neural coupling is thought to play a key role in brain function, as it allows different brain regions to work together in a coordinated manner to process complex information. For example, neural coupling between sensory and motor regions is thought to be important for coordinating movement, while coupling between regions involved in attention and perception is thought to play a role in focusing attention on relevant information.

Neural coupling can also be influenced by various factors, including external stimuli, cognitive tasks, and brain disorders. For example, studies have shown that neural coupling can change in response to exposure to environmental toxins, such as air pollution, and that changes in neural coupling can be associated with various neuropsychiatric disorders, such as schizophrenia.

Neural coupling refers to the coordination of neural activity between different brain regions and is thought to play a key role in brain function and information processing. It represents our intelligence, it represents our incredible capability to parallel computing in our brain and its ability to create, invent, build.

> 2. MIRRORING. Listeners will not only experience the similar brain activity to each other, but also to the speaker.

As we have recently studied in the chapter of Mirrow Neurons, mirroring is a phenomenon in which the neural activity of one person is synchronized with another person. This can occur when two individuals are engaging in a social interaction, such as listening to each other's speech. During a conversation, listeners will often experience similar brain activity to each other, as well as to the speaker, as their brains attempt to match and understand the speech and emotions being expressed.

Studies have shown that this type of neural mirroring can occur between different brain regions, including those involved in language processing, perception, and emotion regulation. For example, when a speaker expresses an emotion, listeners will often experience a similar activation of their own emotion-processing brain regions. This mirroring of neural activity is thought to play a key role in empathy, as it allows us to understand and respond to the emotions of others.

Since the spoken language can lead to mirroring of neural activity, the speaker and listener experience similar brain activity while processing the speech and emotions being expressed. This type of neural mirroring is thought to play a key role in empathy and social interaction.

> 3. DOPAMINE REALEASE. The brain releases dopamine into the system when it experiences an emotionally charged event, making it easier to remember and with greater accuracy.

We already have studied the importance of Dopamine in brain functions, including reward and motivation. When the brain experiences an emotionally charged event, such as a memorable story, it releases dopamine. This improved memory and accuracy in recall of the event.

The release of dopamine in response to emotionally charged events is thought to serve an adaptive function, as it makes it easier for the brain to remember and respond to emotionally significant events. This can be particularly important in the context of storytelling, as an emotionally charged story is more likely to be remembered and retold, allowing important cultural and historical information to be passed down from generation to generation, particularly before the written language.

> 4. CORTEX ACTIVITY. When processing facts, two areas of the brain are activated (Broca's and Wernike's area). A well-told story can engage additional areas, including motor cortex, sensorial cortex, frontal cortex...

Broca's and Wernike's are the key areas. These areas are responsible for processing grammar, syntax, and vocabulary, and are crucial for understanding and producing speech.

However, a well-told story can engage many additional areas. The motor cortex is involved in the control of movement and can be activated when a listener imagines actions being described in the story. The sensory cortex is responsible for processing sensory information, and can be activated when the listener imagines sights, sounds, and other sensory details described in the story. The frontal cortex, which is involved in higher-level cognitive processes such as decision-making and attention, can also be activated as the listener pays attention to and makes sense of the story.

Spoken language can activate a wide range of brain regions, including those involved in processing grammar, syntax, and vocabulary, as well as those involved in imagination, sensory processing, and higher-level cognition. This allows listeners to fully experience and understand the narrative.

SPOKEN LANGUAGE has been crucial in shaping HUMAN CONSCIOUSNESS with an impact on our ability to think, communicate, and understand the world and ourselves in it, that has been crucial in the development of social bonds and cooperation.

It creates our **PRIMARY CONSCIOUSNESS**.

Reason why spoken language build human consciousness is as follows:

1. Communication and social interaction: Spoken language allows us to communicate complex thoughts, ideas, and emotions with others. It facilitates social interaction, cooperation, and the sharing of knowledge and experiences. Through language, we can express our thoughts and feelings, convey information, and engage in meaningful conversations. This ability to communicate and interact with others has played a significant role in the development of human consciousness, as it has allowed for the exchange of ideas and the formation of shared **beliefs and cultural norms**.

2. Abstract thinking and conceptualization: Language enables us to think and express abstract concepts that go beyond immediate sensory experience. Through language, we can conceptualize and discuss ideas, beliefs, values, and hypothetical scenarios. It provides us with a cognitive tool for organizing and structuring our thoughts, allowing us to engage in higher-level thinking processes. Language allows us to create mental representations of the world (we create the world) and to engage in introspection, self-reflection, and metacognition (we create ourselves in the world), which are essential aspects of human consciousness.

3. Memory and knowledge transmission: Spoken language has played a crucial role in the transmission of knowledge and cultural heritage across generations. Through storytelling, oral traditions, and verbal instructions, knowledge and wisdom are passed down from one generation to another. Language allows us to encode, store, and retrieve information, facilitating the accumulation of knowledge over time. This process of **knowledge transmission** has <u>shaped human consciousness</u> by providing a means to learn from the experiences and wisdom of those who came before us.

4. Narrative construction and identity formation: Language allows us to construct narratives about ourselves, others, and the world around us. Through storytelling and language-based narratives, we create meanings, interpret experiences, and form our sense of identity. Language enables us to weave together our personal stories and connect them to broader cultural narratives, influencing our self-perception and understanding of our place in the world. The ability to construct and engage with narratives has been central to the <u>development of human consciousness</u> and our **capacity for self-awareness** in the world.

Overall, spoken language has been crucial in **shaping human consciousness** by enabling communication, abstract thinking, knowledge transmission, and narrative construction. It has provided us with a powerful tool for expressing our thoughts and emotions, engaging in complex cognitive processes, and connecting with others in meaningful ways.

At the beginning it was The WORD, and the word was GOD..., St. Jones 1:1 said in the BIBLE.

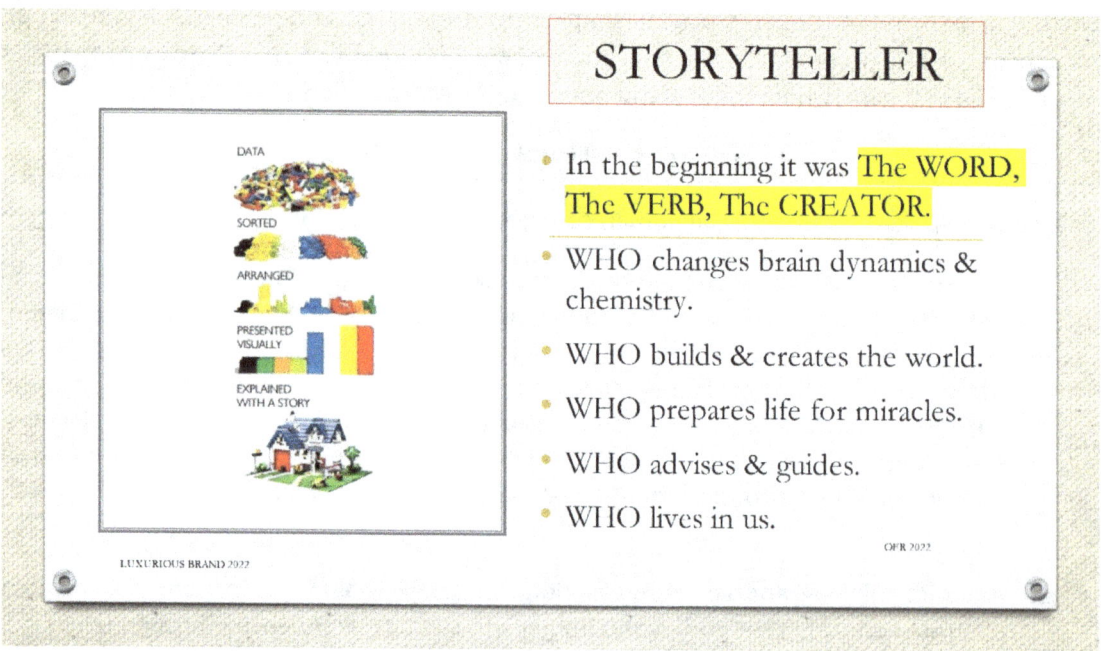

Spoken language had an impact on the way we think and process information. It has allowed us to express and understand abstract concepts, to tell stories and transmit cultural knowledge, and to engage in introspective and self-referential processing in the surrounding world.

On this regard Basque language is a fascinating example. Basque is considered an isolate language with no known relationship to any other language in the world, it comes from the Neolithic period, 10,000 BCE (cave of Ekain, Zestoa in Gipuzkoa, with cultural and artistic manifestations), period in which agriculture started to develop human settlements. One of these settlements was in the Basque region (North of Spain and France), at that time Basque was a spoken language and we cannot demonstrate its exact time of origin since it has no written history of Basque language until the medieval period. Peculiarities of the language are:

1. Ergative-Absolutive Case System, shared by Georgian and indigenous languages of North and Central America. It distinguishes two types of transitive verbs: those with direct object (absolutive) and those with a subject complement (ergative). It makes clear who is important and who is doing what.

2. Polysynthetic: It creates very long words by gluing different morphemes (the smallest units of meaning in a language). This makes words long and complex. It is shared by the indigenous languages of North and Central America, such as Navajo and Mohawk. Polysyntheses is developed in communities where close observation of natural world and environment is essential for survival and requires economy to express situations. Linguistics are studying polysynthetic languages to understand how they develop and change over time, and how they reflect the culture and way of life of the people.

3. Agglutinative: Words are formed by adding affixes to a root word. This gives flexibility in formation but also complexity. Represents an economy of expression of complex ideas and relationships, particularly social relationship and status. Example of agglutinative languages are: Turkish, Japanese, Swahili, Hungarian.

4. Verb Initial, VSO language: Sentences begin with the verb, therefore emphasize the action or the event. Verb-Subject-Object (VSO) languages are Classical Arabic, Welsh, and Tagalog.

5. **Complex Phonology:** It has a large number of consonants not found in other languages, a unique vowel system, and unique sounds i.e. set of consonants known as "ejectives," produced with a burst of air from the glottis. Its rhyme and flow is a way of express meaning and emotions and to influence others. Languages with complex phonology are: Georgian, Taa (Botswana and Namibia),Piraha (Amazonian in Brasil), Arabic (Semitic language).

Ekain cave. Patrimonio De La Humanidad | Ekainberri: Museo de la cueva Ekain, Zestoa, País Vasco

As I explained, verbal languages have a significant impact on how people think, communicate, and understand the world around them. That is probably one of the reasons why I am attracted to languages and one of the reasons why books cannot be literally translated, but have to be rewritten, since language itself impacts brain structure.

Example of social bonds and cooperation in Basque language are:

- Language and Culture: Creating a sense of community and share identity, which has in turn fostered social bonds and cooperation.
- Communication and Understanding: With a unique and complex language with a rich vocabulary and a distinct grammatical structure, to communicate requires a deep understanding of nuances, which foster empathy, understanding, and cooperation.
- Connection to the Land: Many Basque words and phrases relate to the mountains, the sea, and other elements of the natural world. This connection to the land can help to foster a sense of stewardship and respect for the environment, promoting social cooperation and harmony.
- Multilingualism: To foster communication and cooperation across cultures they require to be multilingual (Spanish, French, English)

Comparable influences can be seen in other regional languages or dialects all over the world.

WRITTEN LANGUAGE

WRITTEN LANGUAGE is another story. What we described above (WE inside the world around us) does not happen in written language. Written language, on the contrary, was able to modify our ancestors "primary consciousness", by impacting the brain **Default Mode Network (DMN)** (the "me center" in the brain) and producing a crucial leap. Witten language was able to transform their internal voices from non-personal (a hallucination as in schizophrenia or dreaming) towards our existing "SECONDARY CONSCIOUSNESS" controlled abstractly by creating a representation of ourselves, of our BEING and recognizing the inner voice as our own (as in the Lucid Dreams).

Hughe improvement in the evolution of Human Beings, that will require in the future another upgrade to hear the inner voice of others (telepathy) and to accept our Liberation assuming our Trinity (Mind-Body-Soul) our world creative activity.

Humans are the only species capable to produce and understand complex speech (animals might have some limited abilities). Language (the WORD) is a defining characteristic of the human mind and does play a significant role in shaping our perceptions and understanding and creating the REALITY.

LANGUAGE is for human mind the Prime Reactivity, the ULTIMATE REALITY. It allows us to communicate abstract concepts, create narratives, and build complex societies.

<mark>We act as the creators of the reality.</mark>

POETRY (logos, words) is a step further, a primary activity of the INFINITE CONSCIOUSNESS. Poetry does not describe objects, it just uses language to take the same pathway that trace us into The Source, into the Ultimate Reality, into Allah, into God... Poetry is indeed an art form that uses language in a unique and expressive way, often exploring abstract concepts and emotions that are difficult to put into words. For some people, poetry can serve as a tool for connecting with a higher power or a sense of the divine.

If you are good dominating language, words, intonation, it means that you are close to THE SOURCE (to your God...). Your body is blessed by HIM, the humility of your soul is chosen to show how **to create** the reality.

Be proud to accept what **He** offers you

Multiply it and let it build a reality by its own.

You are now a world creator.

Take the task to codify God languages into a wonderful reality storytelling. **It comes from your inside** after meeting your consciousness and it is given to the world in Infinite Deep Experiences to bring our happiness to return into the Ultimate Reality.

Be blessed in every experience. Go to the reality we share with everyone and everything. **Feel the gap** of how people see his body and perceive the world. **Accomplish the circle** of life, return to your ULTIMATE HAPPINESS.

Feel full, feel empowered, feel a warrior, raise the consciousness, feel guided by your Angels, feel solid in your dream. **Be happy building** your story, creating your world, go deeply into the content of experience.

Live in the Deep Intuition because the awareness that you have is the Deep Reality of the world.

Become a world creator. Create the world you would love to live in.

Through writing, people have been able to record their thoughts, experiences, and knowledge, and pass them down from generation to generation. This has allowed us to build upon the accumulated wisdom of the past and to advance our understanding of the world and ourselves.

The written language has also been instrumental in shaping HUMAN CONSCIOUNESS by providing a permanent record of our thoughts and experiences. It has allowed us to reflect upon them and to develop a more abstract understanding of ourselves and the world around us. This shift from a non-personal to personal and abstract understanding of consciousness has been referred to as the transformation from primary to secondary consciousness.

The DMN-Default Mode Network, plays a role in self-referential and introspective processing, reflecting on our thoughts and feelings. The development of writing and the subsequent shift towards secondary consciousness changed DMN activity, allowing us to better control our inner voice and to recognize it as our own. This not only allowed us to better understand ourselves and the world, but also to communicate our thoughts and experiences to others.

WRITTEN LANGUAGE has played a direct role in shaping our SECONDARY CONSCIOUSNESS changing our DMN or Brain Default Mode Network our "me center" to better understanding ourselves.

This is in fact the main reason of this book, to elevate our Secondary Consciousness into the INFINITE CONSCIOUSNESS, to understand and live our Trinity and gain our LIBERATION.

Both written and spoken language are closely intertwined and have likely influenced each other throughout human history. While written language has allowed us to create a permanent record of our thoughts and experiences, spoken language has allowed us to communicate these in real-time and to engage in face-to-face communication.

Written and spoken language has been crucial in shaping human consciousness (Primary and Secondary) with similar impact on our ability to think, communicate, understand and create both the world and ourselves.

The transition from primary to secondary consciousness is believed to have occurred with the development of complex language, particularly written language. Language allowed individuals to create an **internal dialogue** and engage in abstract thought, introspection, and the representation of the self. This development enabled individuals to have a more sophisticated understanding of their own thoughts and experiences, leading to the emergence of a SECONDARY CONSCIOUSNESS.

While primary consciousness is characterized by immediate sensory experiences and instinctual responses, the secondary consciousness involves higher-level cognitive processes, abstract thinking, self-reflection, and the ability to represent and understand one's own mental states. The development of complex language played a significant role in the transition from primary to secondary consciousness.

These concepts of primary and secondary consciousness are based on the work of Julian Jaynes, a psychologist and philosopher.

❑ Primary Consciousness: refers to a state of awareness characterized by direct sensory experiences and immediate emotional responses. It is associated with the present moment and the here-and-now. Primary consciousness is thought to be more prevalent in early human civilizations and in non-human animals. It involves basic perceptual awareness, basic emotions, and instinctual responses. In this state, individuals may have a limited sense of self-awareness and rely primarily on sensory input and **instinctual behavior**.

❑ Secondary Consciousness: also known as reflective consciousness, represents a more complex form of awareness. It involves the ability to **think about one's own** thoughts, feelings, and experiences. Secondary consciousness allows individuals to reflect on the past, anticipate the future, and engage in abstract thinking, introspection, and self-awareness. It enables individuals to have a sense of personal identity, engage in self-reflection, and make deliberate decisions based on internal mental processes. But remember, regardless they do not write, animals able to dream possess a Phenomenological Consciousness and can create a more or less elaborated moral reasonings as we will study in our second book.

The existence of a Dual Consciousness evolution explains why good scripts (essentially written language) has to clearly show our secondary consciousness, our inner thoughts and representations, leaving the primary consciousness representation, the instinct behavior, to actor's ability.

According to the modern theories of Jacques Lacan, human subject is fundamentally split in two, with their "conscious mind" constantly seeking to reconcile through "the language". The relationship between language and the self, creates and shapes HUMAN SUBJECTIVITY (in the sense that we create our own world). The symbolic order (WORD) containing social norms, values, and institutions, gives us a structure for our interactions with the world and with others. This limits our ability to fully express our desires and our unconscious mind. That tension between unconscious impulses and the symbolic order creates in the individual, a sense of dissatisfaction or lack, leading to continually seek to fill this void through various means, such as consumer culture, sex, or power... Lacan's ideas about the relationship between desire and the symbolic order have implications for ethics and politics. He argues that in contemporary society, there is a tendency to the ==hypertrophy or overemphasize ethics== at the expense of politics. This means that political issues are transformed into mere individual ethical issues, thus rendering them less collective and more personal. Our continuous seeking of pleasure results in that political ideas or thoughts are accepted only when they produce us pleasure, regardless any objective analysis. This allow you to understand that we are guided by a dopamine life, creating dependency and justifying fanatism, populism and any type of extremisms. See also the CULTURAL CONDITIONING and the DOPAMIN PLAY section.

Another peculiarity of "the WORD/the VERB of Human Beings" is their **TEACHING IMPULSE**. Learning is common in all animals, but the strong pulsion to teach/share is idiosyncratic in humans. It explains the endless need to know and consolidate what is learned (*docendo discimus*) and to forge the THEORY OF MIND of oneself and the others building our **Personal consciousness**, studied in chapter two.

If I write a book, the main reason is to teach, in this case the TRILOGY of the HUMAN BEING, to convince myself and you on what I shared. In other words, it is a way to build my own Personal Consciousness, and a way to assure that my mind and yours could communicate and have commonalities. To assure that some of you can share with me the Ultimate Consciousness and that both understand that we are one in God, whatever this God can be… My teaching instinct has been forged more than 60 years, now it is time to demonstrate myself and to you that is a good one.

I know that the most effective teaching is storytelling building. This book has some principles and priorities, anatomical and medical knowledge, but particularly is built with narratives, to capture your mind, to let you think. My understanding on the topic is not enough profound to be able to build paroles, I am a student like you. But I want to share it in order you be able to perfectionate when it grows in your Personal Consciousness. Whatever you discover, whatever you understand please let me know. I will love to share it.

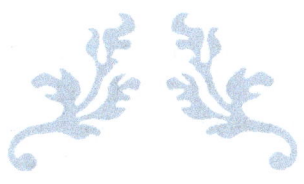

THE EGO

The EGO plays a significant role in human conduct. It is the part of our psyche that mediates between the conscious and unconscious mind, and it is responsible for our sense of self-identity. The EGO is often associated with our sense of self-importance and self-esteem, and it can influence our behavior in both positive and negative ways.

A **Healthy EGO**, what we use to call the **"BEING"**, can help us set realistic goals, make good decisions, and be assertive when necessary. It can also help us to maintain our self-esteem and self-worth, which is important for overall well-being.

An **unhealthy EGO** or overdeveloped EGO that we refer as **"EGO"** can lead to negative behaviors such as narcissism, arrogance, and manipulation. It can also lead to an inflated sense of self-importance, which can cause us to disregard the needs and feelings of others. In extreme cases, an unhealthy EGO can lead to a pathological sense of self, where a person's sense of self becomes so distorted that they have difficulty functioning in their everyday lives.

The "EGO-related disorders" are personality disorders associated with excessive focus on the self and an inflated sense of self-importance such as:

- Narcissistic Personality Disorder: characterized by an inflated sense of self-importance, a strong need for admiration, and a lack of empathy for others.
- Histrionic Personality Disorder: characterized by excessive attention-seeking behavior, an exaggerated sense of self-importance, and a need for approval and attention from others.
- Borderline Personality Disorder: characterized by unstable and intense relationships, impulsive behavior, and an unstable sense of self-identity.
- Antisocial Personality Disorder (formerly referred to as psychopathy/sociopathy): have a persistent pattern of antisocial behavior, impaired empathy and remorse, and egotistical and manipulative tendencies (25% inmates in jail belong to this group). Specifically, have
  1. Lack of empathy or concern for others
  2. Impulsiveness and risk-taking behavior
  3. Deceitfulness and manipulation
  4. Lack of guilt or remorse
  5. Aggressive or violent behavior
  6. Irresponsible behavior and a disregard for obligations and rules
  7. Difficulty forming and maintaining relationships.
  8. Superficial charm and charisma
  9. Grandiose sense of self-worth

It is obvious that many of this EGO-related disorders are related with neurotransmitter disfunction.

- ➤ **Serotonin**: High levels of serotonin increase self-stem and social dominance, which could potentially contribute to dictatorial behavior.
- ➤ **Dopamine**: High levels of dopamine have increased sensation-seeking behavior, impulsivity, and risk-taking. Individuals with a genetic variation that enhances dopamine function may be more likely to exhibit traits associated with psychopathy, such as lack of empathy and manipulative behavior.

> ➤ **Oxytocin**: In charge of prosocial behavior, may also contribute to ingroup favoritism and <u>outgroup hostility</u>, with manipulative behavior towards certain groups.

The EGO plays a crucial role in human conduct influencing our behavior in both positive and negative ways. It is important for individuals to be aware of the role of the EGO in their lives and to strive for a balance between a healthy sense of self and humility. A positive BEING that we use to recognized as a GOOD PERSON.

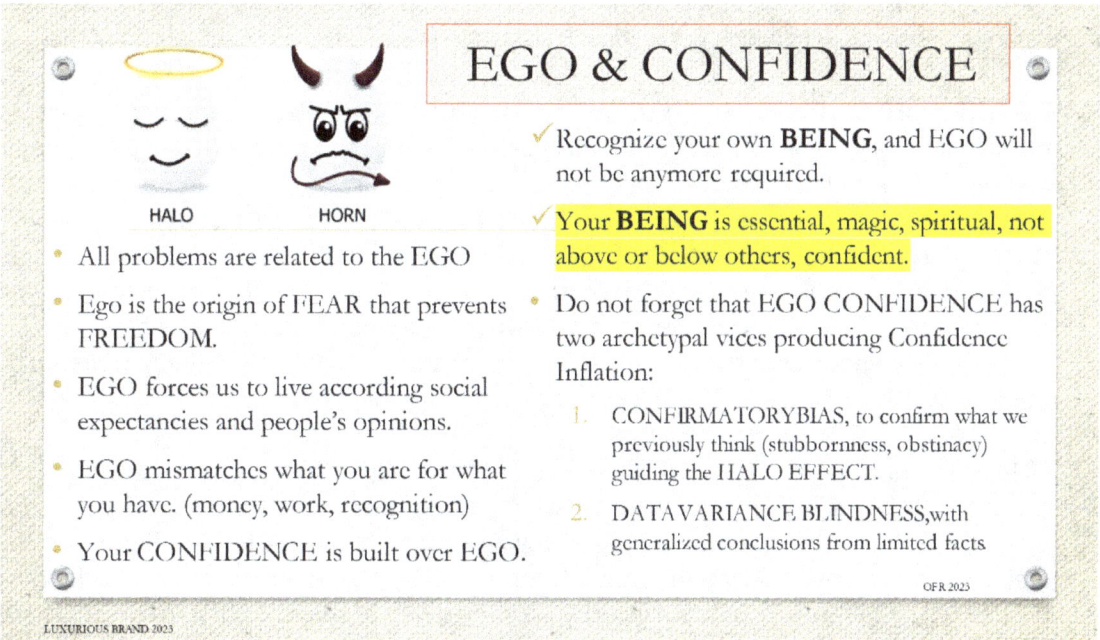

EGO & CONFIDENCE

HALO   HORN

- All problems are related to the EGO
- Ego is the origin of FEAR that prevents FREEDOM.
- EGO forces us to live according social expectancies and people's opinions.
- EGO mismatches what you are for what you have. (money, work, recognition)
- Your CONFIDENCE is built over EGO.

✓ Recognize your own **BEING**, and EGO will not be anymore required.

✓ Your **BEING** is essential, magic, spiritual, not above or below others, confident.

- Do not forget that EGO CONFIDENCE has two archetypal vices producing Confidence Inflation:
  1. CONFIRMATORY BIAS, to confirm what we previously think (stubbornness, obstinacy) guiding the HALO EFFECT.
  2. DATA VARIANCE BLINDNESS, with generalized conclusions from limited facts.

OFR 2023

LUXURIOUS BRAND 2023

We are HUMAN BEINGS; we carry our Trinity inside.

A GOOD PERSON

It might be possible that you have ask yourself what a good person is, how can I identify a good person, or even how can I be a good person. Regardless the fact that solitary people have a well develop 6th sense (intuition) to detect PEOPLE'S VIBRATION and spontaneously recognized who is good and who is bad, there are a series of facts that immediately allow you to recognize a good person. This are: **benevolence, conformity,** and **traditionalism**. Maybe it sounds to you estrange but you will understand it immediately. Added to this top three, they also have **sincerity** and **humility**.

- **BENEVOLENCE**: A good person is characterized by **seeking the well-being of the people** with whom he has contact. Thus, the benevolent person can leave the bubble of "the self" to think about others, their well-being, their quality of life and their needs. Benevolence is important not only for our everyday interpersonal relationships, but also for society in general. The human disposition to be benevolent is essential to our nature and is the foundation for life in society. So, if we want to be good people, we must begin to cultivate benevolence in our daily lives.

- **CONFORMITY:** When we say that good people is conform, we do not mean that they are conformists or that they simply conform to the opinions of the group. We refer to the ability they have to moderate their actions, inclinations, and impulses so as **not to offend or harm others** or violate social expectations or norms. The moderation of the good person is manifested in their actions and in their relationship with pleasures. The moderate man is not moderate in all appetites, but in regard to the objects of some senses such as taste and touch. Moderation leads people to avoid extremes and to maintain a balance in their actions. And particularly being very sensitive not to take part in confrontations linked to emotions or strong feelings (war, religion, political parties, personal integrity...) in which both sides have strong reasons to fight for their opinions.

- **TRADITIONALISM:** Traditionalism is defined as **respect, commitment and acceptance** of the customs and ideas proposed by the cultural tradition. Good people have a deep respect for the cultural customs under which they have grown up. Their commitment to their culture leads them to always seek the best for it. Therefore, these types of people respect tradition. But what is tradition? Basically, it is a social construction that changes temporarily from one generation to another. Tradition varies within each culture, over time and according to social groups, and between different cultures. The good person knows how to understand these changes, accepts them, and commits to them in **search of the best**.

- **SINCERITY:** Sincerity is another of the traits of good people. Although they are not only sincere, but they are also very **empathic when telling the truth**. There are many sincere people, but many are in a rude and hurtful way. Good people are not indifferent to the feelings they arouse by telling the truth. Therefore, they are very careful not to offend or hurt by telling the truth. After all, sincerity expresses with absolute truth and assertiveness what it feels and what it is. It is an important value, since through it you can have better relationships, **respecting others and oneself**.

- **HUMILITY:** Good people are humble. They never feel superior to others and will not look down on them. They recognize that everyone has their own projects and goals, therefore, they respect the success of others and do not get in the way of it. **Humility leads to simplicity**. Therefore, people who choose **kindness**, enjoy the little things in life and the company of their loved ones. They value that in the simplicity of life where happiness and peacefulness are found.

We have already treated some drawbacks of the Conformity and Traditionalism in the chapter Does EVIL exist? when we talked about SOCIAL CONDICIONALISM and how it can shape our neuronal circuits to extreme level of fanaticism, fundamentalism, terrorism... also studied in the DOPAMINE PLAY section.

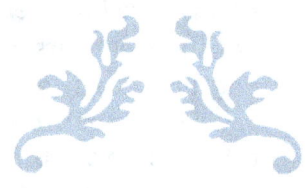

PEOPLE'S VIBRATION

If we could recognize and use our intuition to detect people's vibration things will be much simpler.

David R. Hawkins developed a "map of consciousness" based on the concept of vibrations. He believed that emotions could be classified as having different vibrational frequencies, with negative emotions (such as fear, anger, and guilt) having low frequencies and positive emotions (such as love, joy, and peace) having high frequencies. According to Hawkins, people who primarily experience low frequency emotions are in a state of "survival consciousness," while those who experience high frequency emotions are in a state of "power consciousness."

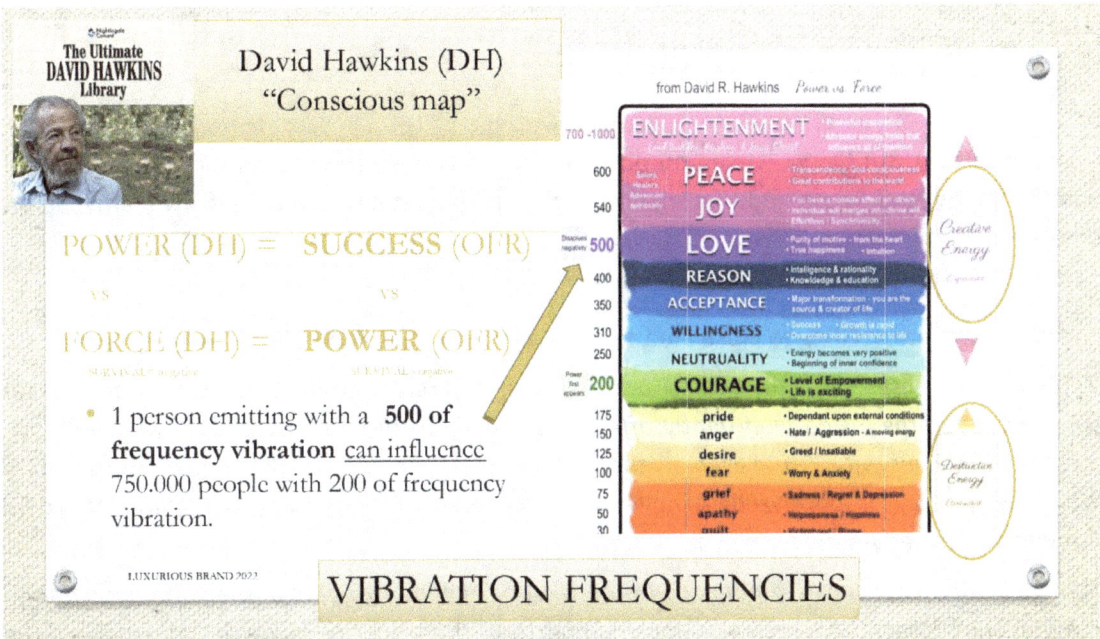

In contrast to David Hawkins' nomenclature that classify as "Force" the negative emotions of people with low vibrations expressing exclusive survival feelings, and as "Power" the high vibrational people, we consider the Power to be negative and the Success to be their positive counterpart.

The reason has already been introduced in the chapter of positivity. For us is much closer to the reality to consider that **POWER** is based on a **negative perception** of fear, on the **HARM** you could produce, including the limitation/control of people's freedom and free will and mind influence on others.

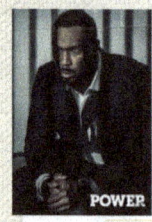
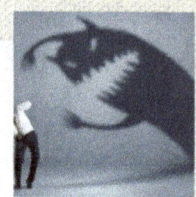

YOUR POWER

- Your POWER depend on the number and the **type of ALLIANCES** you can engage near you.

- And the effect this alliances will have in the ability or the freedom of your peers

- And how effective this alliances will be in directly creating disgust and rejection about the results of your opponents.

- POWER refers to the SOCIAL power, and the **FEAR** other people view in you for whatever reason.

- ==POWER is based on **negative perception** on the **HARM** you could produce==, including the limitation/control of people's freedom and free will and mind influence on others.

- In the conscious map of David Howkins it is named as "The FORCE" (next slide), naming the Success as "The POWER" which is very confusing.

LUXURIOUS BRAND 2022

China's Biggest Movie Star Was Erased From the Internet, and the Mystery Is Why   - WSJ

On the contrary, **SUCCESS** is based on positive emotions of respect-admiration-love obtained with Empathy and Trust, fighting against our survival primitive and negative amygdala's emotions.

There is a nice storytelling to illustrate the importance to build RESPECT:

*When a **WOLF loses the fight** against another wolf and understands that he no longer has a chance to win, the losing wolf gently offers the jugular to the opponent, as if to say "I lost, let's get this over with." However, in that moment the incredible takes place. The winning wolf, inexplicably, is paralyzed. A millenary force prevents him from killing the one who humbly acknowledges defeat.*

Some primary mechanism, embedded in the DNA or beyond, triggers in the winning wolf and reminds him that <u>the species is more important </u>than the pleasure of eliminating the opponent. What a wonderful instinctive watchmaking! They RESPECT each other. No one would call the wolf who surrenders a coward, or the one who is paralyzed commiserating, the miracle just happens. Neither winner nor defeated.

*Both wolves drift away, and **the wheel of life continues**. And this is known as: HUMILITY.*

> "We make a living by what we get, but we make a life by what we give"
>
> Winston Churchill.

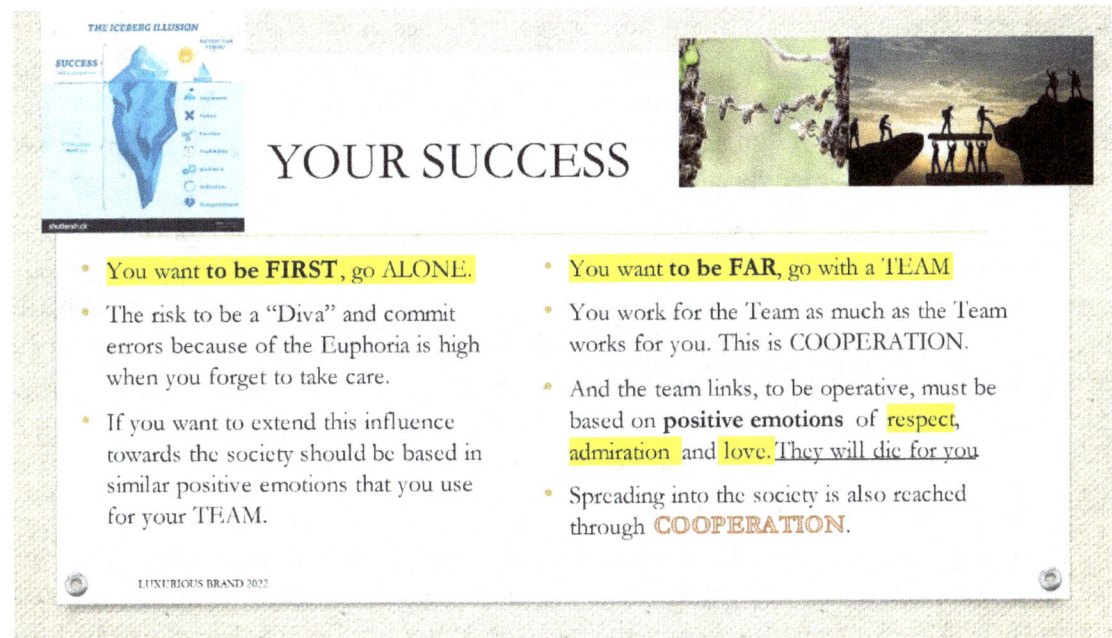

YOUR SUCCESS

- You want **to be FIRST**, go ALONE.
- The risk to be a "Diva" and commit errors because of the Euphoria is high when you forget to take care.
- If you want to extend this influence towards the society should be based in similar positive emotions that you use for your TEAM.

- You want **to be FAR**, go with a TEAM
- You work for the Team as much as the Team works for you. This is COOPERATION.
- And the team links, to be operative, must be based on **positive emotions** of respect, admiration and love. They will die for you
- Spreading into the society is also reached through COOPERATION.

LUXURIOUS BRAND 2022

The most important emotion for success is subjective and can vary depending on the individual and their goals. However, it is commonly suggested that a positive attitude, self-confidence, and resilience are important emotions for success. These emotions can help individuals overcome obstacles, stay motivated, and maintain a growth mindset. Additionally, having a sense of purpose and drive, as well as being able to effectively manage stress, can also contribute to success.

> Does your achievements contribute to a goal that is bigger than you?

Vibrations can stimulate nerve endings in the skin, which can then activate neural pathways that lead to the release of neurotransmitters. For example, vibrations at specific frequencies have been shown to activate the release of serotonin. For example, whole-body vibration at a frequency of 25 Hz was associated with an increase in serotonin levels in rats. Other studies have used lower frequency vibrations, such as 10 Hz or below, and have reported similar effects. Additionally, certain types of body vibrations, such as those generated by exercise or massage, can stimulate the release of endorphins, which are neurotransmitters that are associated with pain relief and feelings of pleasure. Low-frequency sound at 25 Hz has been explored as a possible treatment for a variety of conditions, including pain, inflammation, and osteoporosis. The lower level of human hearing is around 20 Hz.

We are part of the physical law of the resonance, and that include synchronization. Everyone is aware that when several women work closely together, the menstrual period date is synchronized in all of them. We already mention in the hypnosis chapter the high level of electrical brain wave synchronization in efficient working teams. And furthermore, there is the phenomena of INTERPERSONAL SYNCHRONY related with the Mirrow Neurons by which some person actions alter the behavior of others creating a feel of empathy from the Prefrontal Cortex (PFC) to the amygdala and a synchronous behavior. The PFC coordinates the emotional response.

This let you know that your vibrations have a clear influence in your surroundings. But what you maybe do not realize is that it also has an influence in yourself. Let me explain it, your own facial expressions (serious, smile, frowning face …) do have a direct influence on the affective component of your humor response. This indicates that people's facial expressions influence their affective experiences.

It is the so-called **Facial Feedback** hypothesis postulated by Darwin in the XIX century. Our own facial expression alters our hedonic evaluation and modify our own autonomous nervous system (heart rate, skin conductance, skin temperature, blood volume…) The facial feedback hypothesis proposes that facial expressions can influence and even generate corresponding emotions. It suggests that the muscle movements involved in making a particular facial expression can trigger the associated emotional state. For example, smiling can generate a feeling of happiness, while frowning can generate a feeling of sadness.

Mechanisms to explain this effect include:

1. Feedback from the facial muscles to the brain. This feedback can influence the brain's emotional processing centers, resulting in changes to emotional experiences. For example, when a person smiles, the movement of the facial muscles sends signals to the brain that are associated with positive emotions, which can enhance the experience of happiness.
2. Social signaling function of facial expressions. Facial expressions are a primary means of communicating emotions to others, and the display of certain facial expressions can elicit corresponding emotional responses in others. For example, when a person sees someone else smiling, they may feel happier themselves. This social signaling function can also influence a person's own emotional state, as their own facial expressions can signal to themselves the appropriate emotion to feel in a given situation.

In summary, the human body is subject to the physical law of resonance, which states that a system will respond most strongly to a stimulus at its natural frequency. In other words that the rate of the vibration projected, will harmonize with and attract back energies with the same resonance. This is where **the Law of Attraction** comes into play. How we allow ourselves to feel, and how we speak to ourselves will become our physical reality. We produce our own miracles.

> We attract, we create our physical reality. We are the builders of our world.

Whatever you project is whatever you get. This is the Karma law with the 12 principles

1. The Cause-Effect law. What you give is what you get and the rest of the laws are consequence of this one.
2. The Creation law. You are the co-creator of your life, your destiny, your future. Nothing is by chance.
3. The Humble law. Be humble to accept that whatever is in your life derive from your pass actions.
4. The Growth Law. Everything starts and ends in you. You are the alfa and the omega.
5. The Responsibility Law. Be responsible of what are at your surroundings (actions, thoughts, your life in general)
6. The Connection Law. Your past is related with your present and your future. No action is disconnected.
7. The Focus Law. To get important results does not do too many things at the same time.

8. The Generosity Law. Maintain the equilibrium between what to think and what to do. You must practice what you believe in and do it often.
9. The Here and Now Law. Your life is the Present, here and now.
10. The Change Law. The universe explain you several times what has to change.
11. The Patience Law. Wait with patience and serenity for the reward.
12. The Importance Law. It preaches the importance of individual contributions in the sum of a group whole.

This means that the human body can resonate or vibrate in response to external stimuli, such as sound or vibrations not only in the environment but inside us. In terms of synchronization with other bodies, it is possible for the vibrations or movements of one person to influence and synchronize with those of another person. This phenomenon, known as ENTRAINMENT, is seen in various contexts, including music, dance, and even speech. For example, when people dance together to the same rhythm, their movements may become synchronized, leading to a sense of unity and coordination. Similarly, when people speak together, their speech patterns may become synchronized, leading to a more harmonious and coordinated conversation.

This synchronization between bodies can occur at both the conscious and unconscious levels and is thought to be influenced by factors such as social context, cultural norms, and personal relationships.

CLOSING THE EGO

Having studied the relevance of the Ego, you might question yourself if topics covered in this book are written guided by the EGO, or they are a manifestation from a confident BEING. The intention was to belong to the BEING TRINITY, but it is obvious that they can carry the "confirmatory bias" and a "variance blindness".

They are written following the internal voice hoping to be the HUMAN BEING TRINITY but could also just be the EGO. The ego is often associated with certain vices or negative traits, such as pride, arrogance, and a lack of humility. These vices can lead to a confirmation bias, which is the tendency to seek out and interpret information in a way that confirms one's preexisting beliefs or hypotheses. This can lead to a closed-mindedness and resistance to new ideas or perspectives.

The variation bias is the tendency to overestimate the amount of variation or difference in a situation, leading to a belief that things are more unique or special than they really are. This can lead to a lack of perspective and an inability to see commonalities or patterns in the world.

Both biases are often associated with the ego, as they both stem from a self-centered perspective and a lack of humility. They can both lead to a distorted view of reality and can make it difficult for individuals to make accurate assessments or decisions.

Confidence without Ego (meaning the Being) can help counteract the previous biases by allowing an individual to approach situations and information objectively, rather than being influenced by their own biases and preconceptions. When an individual has confidence in their abilities and knowledge, they are more likely to be open to new ideas and perspectives, and less likely to be swayed by their own biases.

To counter the confirmation bias, a person with confidence without ego (the Human Being) can actively seek out information and perspectives that challenge their own beliefs and be willing to change their mind when presented with new evidence. They can also be more aware of their own biases and actively work to overcome them.

To counter the variation bias, a person with confidence without ego (the Being) can approach new situations and people with a sense of curiosity and openness, rather than immediately jumping to conclusions about their uniqueness or specialness. They can also strive to see the commonalities and patterns in the world, rather than focusing solely on the differences.

Ultimately, having confidence without ego, behaving as a Human Beings, means having a sense of self-assurance that is not tied to one's own ego and self-importance, but rather to one's own abilities and knowledge. This can allow individuals to approach situations and information objectively and make better decisions.

It seems obvious that the approach in the book is subjective, regardless the medical, pathologic, psychiatric, religious, and social experiences accumulated in hundreds of travels all over the world and in millions of people interactions. But despite the hundred books read this is a spiritual and moral perception of the self-identity that is supposed to be built upon the feelings of BEING but that could come from the feel of EGO.

No way to demonstrate, it is true for me and if it became also true for the readers this will mean that has overcome the confirmation bias and the variation bias and therefore that is closer to the BEING then to the EGO. Readers, your feed-back is appreciated.

I am suggesting that if readers can see truth in the statement, despite it challenges their own beliefs or biases, it is a sign that they are less likely to be influenced by confirmation bias. And if an individual can see commonalities in a statement rather than focusing on differences, it is a sign that they are less likely to be influenced by variation bias.

However, it is important to note that it is not possible to fully eliminate confirmation bias and variation bias, as they are natural human cognitive biases that everyone is susceptible to. Additionally, the idea that "being" is separate and distinct from the ego is a philosophical concept, and different people may have different ideas about what it means to be in a state of "being."

> BEING is present, is doing, not thinking on what to get/to have but in what to do to serve others.

It is also important to consider that the statement is not a scientific test or a way to measure or demonstrate the truth or the accuracy, but rather a reflection on the relationship between one's own mind and the world.

I wish you can find yourselves, find your true BEING with the help of this book. I will end as I started, we are created to the similarity of God. I admire my perfection as a human being. I realized that we are the Trinity: Mind-Body-Soul.

This book is devoted to show your divinity, to show your Trinity, to gain the Liberation in which Mind, Body and Soul get connected and you finally face the reality of God.

After you understand your TRINITY, you will get convinced that you are never alone.

Your unconsciousness is always with you, guiding you with its INTUITION and your consciousness guiding you with the WORD, and your BODY guided by the Cascade of Consciousness all part of the Infinity Consciousness of GOD.

Just realize that we are limited in our body and what we are looking for is in fact to liberate our Mind and be able to reach through our Soul the Infinity Consciousness. What is that, practical philosophy? Bioethics?

➢ Now is time to build a parable to let you see that the brain is a hardware based system (a machine) not a software based (the consciousness): *My computer is very advanced, I had build in it complex circuits (image recognition, a linear and rotational accelerometer in 3D, …) I stored in it very important documents from me and my surroundings. I discovered and I invented numerous things with my computer and all the data is there. Suddenly one day my computer fail to work, and in spite it was very advanced, it was now too old, so old that I could not find any replacement or spear part. Did I lose everything? Fortunately, no, some of the devices I design in my computer are now working somewhere, and his memory is stored in the cloud with all patents, draws, and software programs.*
Am I lost my work, Am I lost my intelligence? Hopefully no, it is in the cloud.
What can I do? If you trust in your cloud, if your cloud is good, you will be able to access all what you created in another computer. It is not your old computer anymore but is you and your intelligence who is accessible in the cloud. And in the cloud is not only yours but the intelligence of most of us it is the Wisdom of the Universe. Would they going to work in the new-coming outstanding quantum computers in the future. Probably not as it is, but it will update the knowledge, transforming the language in which software was written and will be able to appear again, and show up as coming from you. You will be recognized.

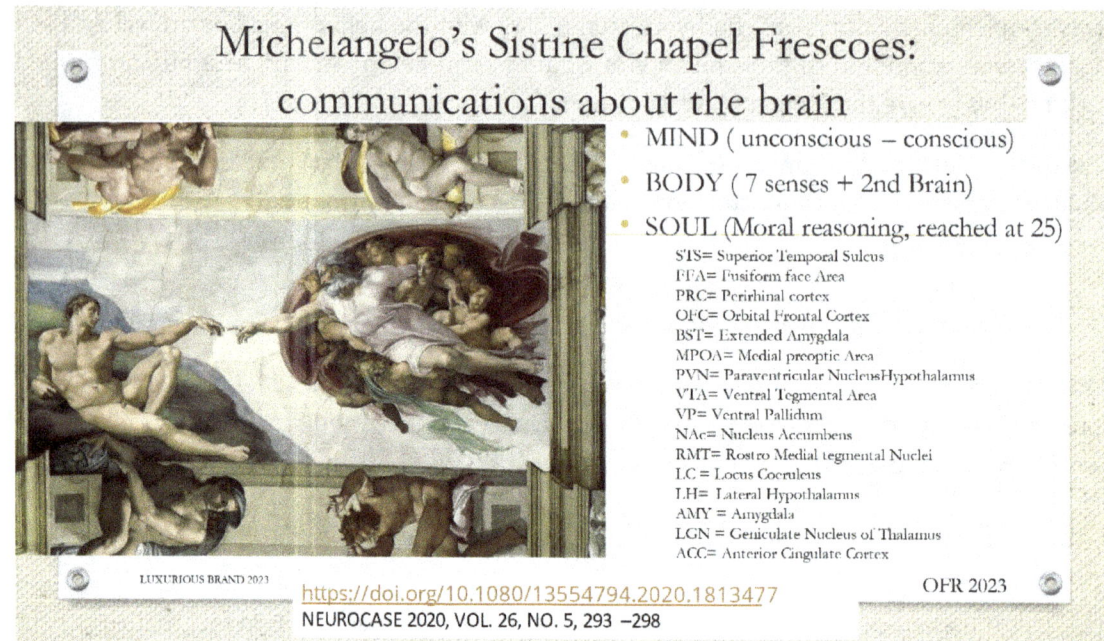

Michelangelo's Sistine Chapel Frescoes: communications about the brain

- MIND (unconscious – conscious)
- BODY (7 senses + 2nd Brain)
- SOUL (Moral reasoning, reached at 25)

STS= Superior Temporal Sulcus
FFA= Fusiform face Area
PRC= Perirhinal cortex
OFC= Orbital Frontal Cortex
BST= Extended Amygdala
MPOA= Medial preoptic Area
PVN= Paraventricular NucleusHypothalamus
VTA= Ventral Tegmental Area
VP= Ventral Pallidum
NAc= Nucleus Accumbens
RMT= Rostro Medial tegmental Nuclei
LC = Locus Coeruleus
LH= Lateral Hypothalamus
AMY = Amygdala
LGN = Geniculate Nucleus of Thalamus
ACC= Anterior Cingulate Cortex

LUXURIOUS BRAND 2023

https://doi.org/10.1080/13554794.2020.1813477
NEUROCASE 2020, VOL. 26, NO. 5, 293 –298

OFR 2023

> It is also time to consider how far away humans had known and have the strong perception that God is within them. We have to address the publication of Wesson Ashford and Brinkley Tatern quoted in the image above and compared this image with the one included in the section Theory of the Mind. In a 1990 the journal of American Medical Association (JAMA) covered the story of Frank Meshberger reporting that Michelangelo's central composition on the Sistine Chapel ceiling (1508–1512), The Creation of Adam, portrays God in the form of a brain. Further, on the front wall of the Sistine Chapel, within the work titled The Last Judgment (1525–1541), the central ellipse, where Jesus is making judgments about good and evil, represents a mid-coronal cross-section of a human brain, implying that the brain is man's instrument for making decisions; In the amygdala were seated two martyrs St. Laurence holding the grate and St. Bartolomew holding his skin in where the self-portrait of Michelangelo Buonarroti can be seen. God is standing up in the Thalamus our central hub of CONSCIOUSNESS as explain in the section about The Intuition Guides you.

Judgments about good and evil

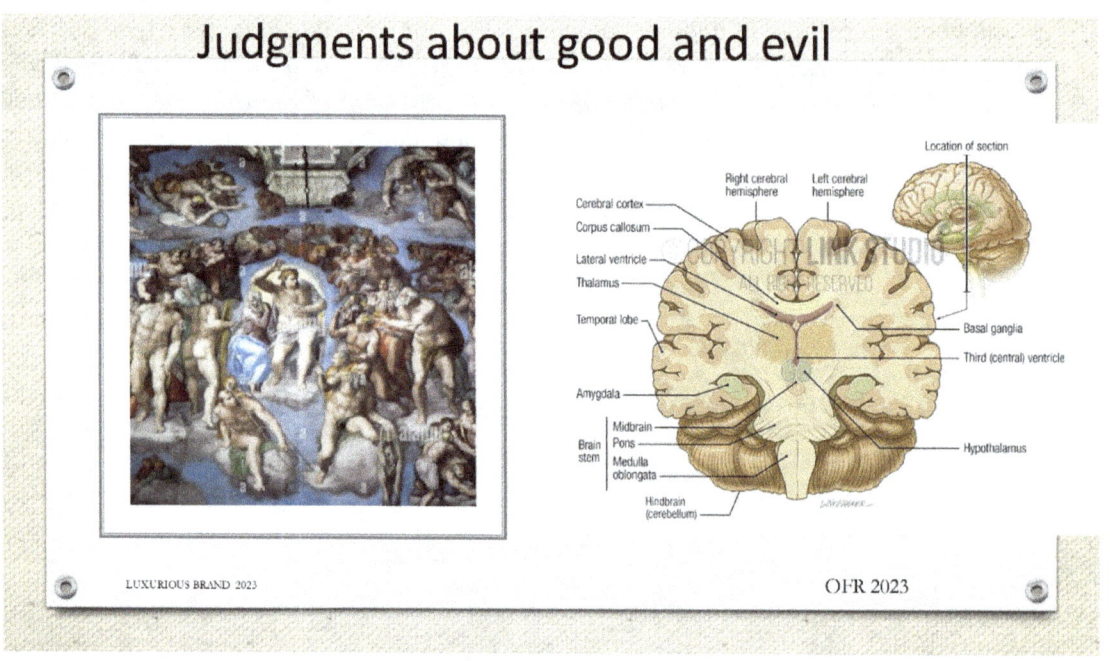

LUXURIOUS BRAND 2023

OFR 2023

Is everything a coincidence, is this by chance?
Remember, our intuition guides us, God is inside us.
We hold the Trinity.

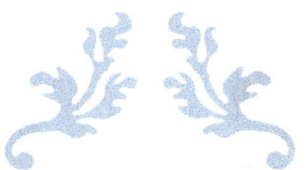

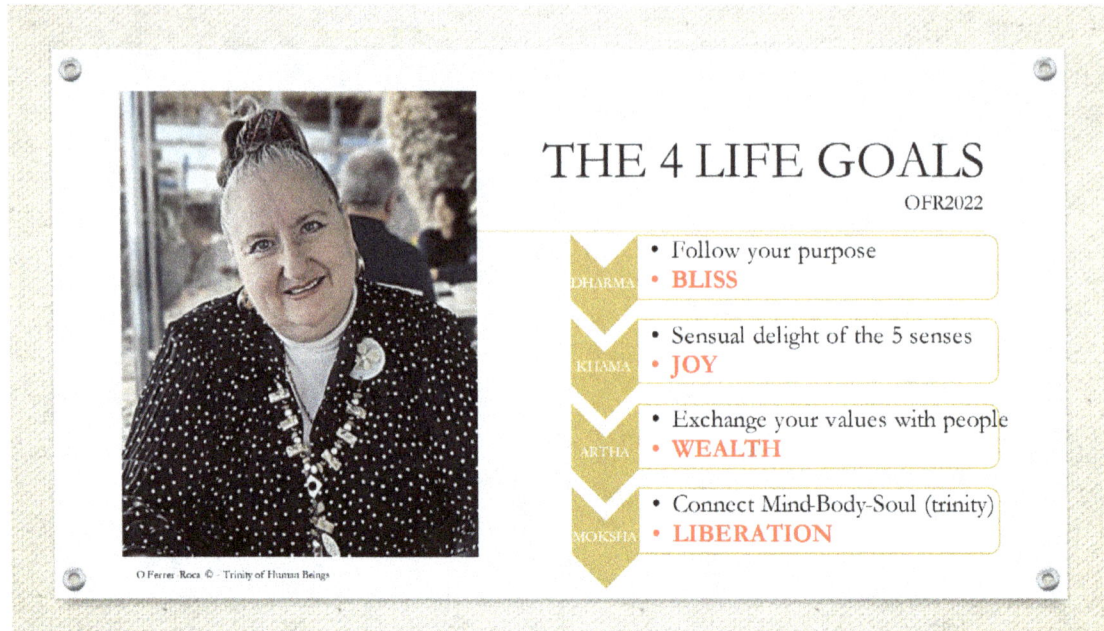

THE 4 LIFE GOALS

OFR2022

DHARMA
- Follow your purpose
- **BLISS**

KHAMA
- Sensual delight of the 5 senses
- **JOY**

ARTHA
- Exchange your values with people
- **WEALTH**

MOKSHA
- Connect Mind-Body-Soul (trinity)
- **LIBERATION**

O Ferrer-Roca © - Trinity of Human Beings

DISCLAIMER

Some of the images used in this book, "TRINITY OF HUMAN BEINGS: The Trinity within, A Journey to understand the Divinity in Ourselves", were obtained from the Internet and have not been authorized or endorsed by the copyright owners to be included in the teaching slides build by the author for didactic purposes and included in the book. Although some slides include the books where they were taken. The author makes no representations or warranties as to the accuracy, completeness or validity of the information contained in the book and accepts no responsibility for the use of any such information. The use of Internet images is solely for the purpose of illustrating the author's ideas and for teaching purposes and does not imply endorsement or affiliation with any entity. Readers are advised to seek their own independent verification of the information contained in the book.

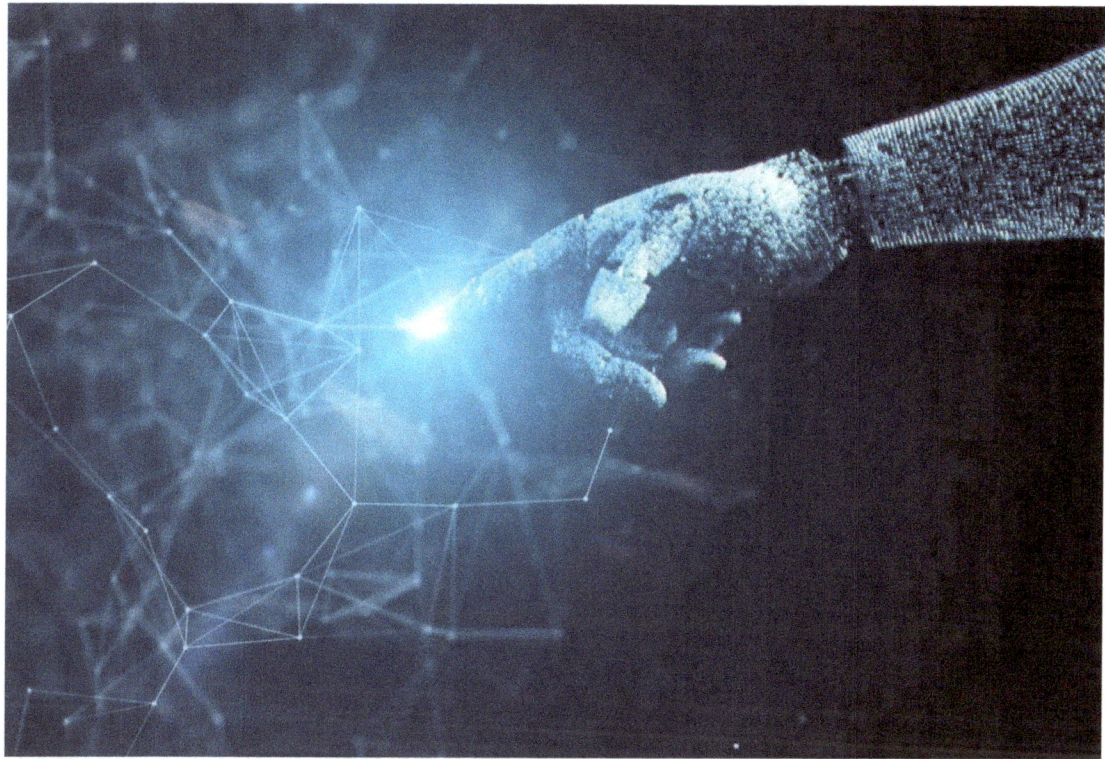

Taken from Forbes.com State-Of-The-Art Applied Artificial Intelligence Defined (forbes.com)

ACKNOWLEDGMENTS

To my parents, to my son, to my pupils, to my friends, to my readers.

Thanks to whom had believed in me and particularly thanks to those who wanted to destroy my life, my work, my carrier. Without them I could never find myself, I could never see my Trinity, I could never get my Liberation.

Not in vain my brain is A Mediator (INFP), someone who possesses the Introverted, Intuitive, Feeling, and Prospecting personality traits. A rare personality type that tends to be quiet, open-minded, and imaginative, and that apply a caring and creative approach to everything I do.